ECOrenaissance

A Lifestyle Guide for Cocreating a Stylish, Sexy, and Sustainable World

Marci Zaroff

Foreword by Horst Rechelbacher

ENLIVEN BOOKS

—

ATRIA

New York   London   Toronto   Sydney   New Delhi

ENLIVEN™

ATRIA

An Imprint of Simon & Schuster, Inc.
1230 Avenue of the Americas
New York, NY 10020

First Enliven Books/Atria Paperback edition August 2018

This publication contains the opinions and ideas of its author. It is intended to provide helpful and informative material on the subjects addressed in the publication. It is sold with the understanding that the author and publisher are not engaged in rendering medical, health, or any other kind of personal professional services in the book. The reader should consult his or her medical, health, or other competent professional before adopting any of the suggestions in this book or drawing inferences from it.

The author and publisher specifically disclaim all responsibility for any liability, loss, or risk, personal or otherwise, that is incurred as a consequence, directly or indirectly, of the use and application of any of the contents of this book.

For information about special discounts for bulk purchases, please contact Simon & Schuster Special Sales at 1-866-506-1949 or business@simonandschuster.com.

The Simon & Schuster Speakers Bureau can bring authors to your live event. For more information or to book an event, contact the Simon & Schuster Speakers Bureau at 1-866-248-3049 or visit our website at www.simonspeakers.com.

Interior design by Kyoko Watanabe

Manufactured in the United States of America

10 9 8 7 6 5 4 3 2 1

Library of Congress Cataloging-in-Publication Data
Names: Zaroff, Marci, author.
Title: Ecorenaissance : a lifestyle guide for co-creating a stylish, sexy, and sustainable world / Marci Zaroff ; foreword by Horst Rechelbacher.
Description: New York : Atria/Enliven Books, 2018.
Identifiers: LCCN 2017055792 (print) | LCCN 2017059583 (ebook) | ISBN 9781501123610 (ebook) | ISBN 9781501123566 (paperback)
Subjects: LCSH: Environmentalism. | Sustainable living. | Lifestyles—Environmental aspects. | BISAC: HEALTH & FITNESS / Healthy Living.
Classification: LCC GE195 (ebook) | LCC GE195 .Z37 2018 (print) | DDC 640.28/6—dc23
LC record available at https://lccn.loc.gov/2017055792

ISBN 978-1-5011-2356-6
ISBN 978-1-5011-2361-0 (ebook)

This book is dedicated to my late mentor and iconic friend
Horst Rechelbacher
(11/11/41–2/15/14)
Founder, AVEDA Corporation and Intelligent Nutrients

Do you know what you are?

You are a manuscript of a divine letter. You are a mirror reflecting a noble face.

This universe is not outside of you.

Look inside yourself; everything that you want, you are already that.

—Rumi

Contents

7.

Conscious Business and Consumerism • 179

Conclusion • 209

ECOrenaissance

Foreword

Knowing is not enough; we must apply.
Willing is not enough; we must do.
—GOETHE

Dear Reader,

My name is Horst Rechelbacher, and I'm the founder of Intelligent Nutrients and the AVEDA Corporation, both leading environmentally responsible beauty companies.

Since the early 1980s, I have proudly pioneered the market for skin and hair care products derived from organic and natural ingredients, aromatherapy, and the healing power of plants. Throughout my life, I have passionately searched for "renewal" and opportunities for betterment, as I believe that I'm here to serve and inspire others, leveraging the transformational properties of products to effect positive change in the world.

So many of the principles and guidelines running through my life parallel those of Marci's vision of an ECOrenaissance. To me, an ECOrenaissance defines the personal rebirth and reawakening when we consciously decide to grow. This movement is an environmental, yogic, and spiritual journey, recycling our inner wisdom, then projecting it into the world. Through my career, by connecting innovative design, packaging, and technology, I have turned simple visions into realities that touch others in my global community.

I have always realized that to fundamentally flow effortlessly through this rebirth, we must learn not to expect, but instead, to inspect. To live our beliefs. To walk our talk, while exhaling and inhaling—allowing life to be a mantra, a living practice of observation turning into action. In other words, we need to take a perpetual inventory.

The beauty of life is our ability to invent ourselves every day, while serving ourselves, the world around us, and our interconnected ecosystem. Balancing our existence also means facing the dark and addressing it, which ultimately helps us see the light within. We must live "truth," while envisioning and manifesting a new reality.

Business is a vehicle that creates a mutual exchange of trading thoughts and ideas. Whether it is product- or service-driven, that shared "economy" represents an inherent collaboration of energy. For example, even when I started my career as a hairdresser, my providing a haircut conveyed my passion. My client would share in turn with money, and our reciprocal pleasure would function as a powerfully positive whole.

When I founded AVEDA and then Intelligent Nutrients, I learned to create collections comprised of pure energy, made from the love of the plants and the purity of their expression, already programmed to function. These living forces have granted and continue to grant me the opportunity to make a transformational difference. While efforts can sometimes initially appear self-gratifying, they never are. Self is useless without interconnection to others. It's the reflection of self-awareness that matters most.

ECOrenaissance provides a profound blueprint to observe, listen, and then directly plug in to how we deeply feel. Self-examination eventually evolves into team and group observation. Passion and desire to make a difference are the soul and DNA of "oneness," while pure consciousness offers a holistic view of all our dimensions and vibrations.

ECOrenaissance is the focus on people's abilities and, as Marci calls it, "artistic intelligence," constantly evolving and inspiring humanity. Imagine how much closer we will be to God—our truth, our light, our source, and our place in the cosmos—twenty to thirty years from now. This will be the result of our widespread acceptance of a "rebirth."

Be the student, the participant, and the leader. Study cause and effect. Healing is every moment, so it is our conscious choice to turn perception into thought, and belief into action. Let go of the surface to get unstuck. The key is to join the collective. The concept is nothing new; it has just been forgotten by so many. This movement is both essential and eternal. It has always been inside of us. The phone has been ringing, but we've been too preoccupied to pick it up, and it has prevented us from hearing our unified message.

We're unnecessarily learning through crisis and wake-up calls from Mother Earth. She's speaking to us to help us gain clarity of the greater good, our sense of purpose and our global community. More than ever, we're helping others to find their identity through science, media, technology, art, fashion, and business. ECOrenaissance is grounded in spreading the message of how we all benefit from collective action.

An awakening won't come with outward spiritual efforts; we're already spiritual beings within. It will manifest through a divine process. The more we experience, the more we awake. And it must be together, as collaboration is the key to unlocking the door to our abundance. We are one universal village, and there are no borders.

To be truly successful is to be engaged in this reawakening. Reliving the Renaissance is like a reincarnation of our real selves. We're entering a time of activating what already exists. Laws need to be changed to benefit the greater good, not the few. Changing these rules and building a collective consciousness with accountability to the whole should fix what has been broken by corruption and manipulation.

We each must "be the change," as we are the leaders and the instruments. Perhaps more devastating catastrophes will happen because we're so arrogant and need to be humbled. With crisis comes humility, then radical openness, then a real and lasting shift. What happened to kindness? To service? To devotion? From Buddha to Jesus, Gandhi to Martin Luther King Jr., all the great teachers embodied these virtues.

How do we educate? Live it and share it. Work it. Be it.

Exhalation plus inhalation inspire innovation. An equal distribution of heart, energetics, and intuition will lead to this rebirth, to an ECOrenaissance. The necessity for a revolution is upon us, growing with each and every day we take the environment and our humanity for granted. The time is NOW.

I'm happy, really happy. Marci is a conduit of love and light. Like me, she's here to serve and to help usher in the fusion of new and old, tapping the familiar voice of creative vision that threads life and humanity, one cohesive voice for the future. An ECOrenaissance.

Yours in service for a green, healthy, nonviolent planet,

Horst Rechelbacher
(Horst passed away in February 2014, and this was his final writing.)

Introduction

The journey of a thousand miles begins with one step.
—LAO TZU

Not too long ago, I used to have to drive an hour to find the closest health food store or yoga class. The green lifestyle movement was confined to a small, niche community, dismissed by most as crazy hippies and granola-lovers.

While I don't deny my inner tree-hugger, I'm also very much a material girl. I love fashion, travel, and delicious food, and I live in a high-rise in Manhattan. I wasn't raised in a commune, ashram, or a yurt. And I don't grow my own food or climb trees (although it probably would be good for me). So how did I get here?

My journey down the Green Brick Road was a combination of synchronicity and my unquenchable search for more—ideas, innovations, and solutions. It was never about leaving anything behind—it was always about *yes, and.* Looking and feeling fabulous shouldn't come at the expense of living in harmony with the environment—surely I couldn't be the only one who thought this. When I was starting out, though, style and ecology were seen as two dichotomous worlds.

I sought out fashion companies that were forward-thinking, but everything I came across was crunchy, frumpy, boxy, beige, and boring. I drove hours to find organic produce, but the health food stores of the time were limited and cramped. I knew that "green" would never become mainstream if it involved this much sacrifice.

> Looking and feeling fabulous shouldn't come at the expense of living in harmony with the environment.

I felt a deep calling to be part of the solution. If I could take people on a journey where ecology looks, tastes, and feels amazing, I could change the world for the better. I always knew, in my gut, that an ECOrenaissance wasn't an *if*, it was a *when*.

Just over two decades later, I watch in amazement as the world of sustainability continues to transform before my eyes. Once empty environmental business conferences are now sold out. Huge corporations such as Walmart, Costco, and Target are selling more organic produce than Whole Foods, with Amazon now joining the party. Major celebrities are turning the red carpet green with glamorous ECOfashion. CVS and Duane Reade are lining their shelves with natural and organic personal care and beauty products. There is now a widespread acceptance and demand for gorgeous and green.

It's a completely different world, and every single day I wake up and feel like I'm living my dream. And this is just the beginning.

My Journey

Looking back, my journey into the world of ecology and consciousness seems serendipitous. Although I grew up in a sheltered environment in then-rural South Florida (not exactly an eco-centric community), I always hungered for more, for deeper purpose and fulfillment in life. So when inspiration came knocking, I was ready to answer the door.

My initial breakthrough moment came at the age of fifteen. While shopping in the local mall, I encountered a beautiful, somewhat mystical twenty-one-year-old woman named Surya. We struck up a conversation, and there was an inexplicable connection between us, as if we had known each other all our lives. As synchronicity would have it, she worked as a new hairdresser at the salon I had been going to for years. I booked my next appointment with her, and what would follow was a lifelong friendship and mentorship.

Our conversations, delving into everything from food to relationships to spirituality, inspired Surya to offer me one of the most important gifts I'd ever receive, Shakti Gawain's *Living in the Light*. This powerful book struck a profound chord—that there is something more than what we can physically see, so we must listen to and trust our gut, the lifeline to truth. In her book, Shakti states, "Every time you don't follow your inner guidance, you feel a loss of energy, loss of power, a sense of spiritual deadness."[1] This book helped to illuminate the lightbulb within my heart and soul, shining as my compass for the journey ahead.

Surya and I are forever connected. I still remember the day she introduced me to AVEDA clove shampoo, cooked me my first organic plant-based meal, and stood upside down beside me as we learned yoga handstands (before yoga was a widespread concept!). We were in our own little world, our green bubble. And together, we explored and discovered. Every step we took was like opening a new door to an exciting playground of learning and self-discovery.

In 1990, the next auspicious force in my life happened while dining at a macrobiotic restaurant in New York City. While sitting at Ozu on the Upper West Side, I saw a man walk in the door who I thought resembled the renowned artist Peter Max. I was introduced to Peter's art at the age of fifteen, about the same time I met Surya. Betsi, my childhood best friend, had a stepfather who collaborated with Peter at Woodstock and displayed several pieces of his art in their home. I remember how I was drawn to Peter's messaging of "Love," "Peace," and "A Better World," so I began to research his work. The themes in Peter's artwork reflected his life as an environmentalist, vegan, and defender of human and animal rights. He created (and still does) with compassion and purpose, infusing environmental and social commentary into the canvas. I often think of MAX as a modern-day Michelangelo or Da Vinci, using art as a voice for change, a visual journal on the current environmental, political, and societal makeup. Max paints with love and purpose, the elements of ECOrenaissance art.

That day at Ozu, Peter saw me looking at him and asked if he could join me for lunch. I was thrilled. Here was someone whose art had influenced me for years, driving me further toward a creative and conscious lifestyle. And now there he was standing before me, in my favorite restaurant, asking to sit with me. Pinching myself, we explored ideas over tempeh, kale, and hijiki.

In 1990, inspired by *Gulliver's Travels*, I had conceived of starting a holistic health school called Gulliver's Living & Learning Center—dedicated to taking people on a journey to the lands of health, environmental wellness, and self-realization. As I shared my vision with Peter, he immediately responded by offering his support. He designed my first logo and business card for the school. And his art appeared on the cover and launch issue of our magazine, *Macrocosm*, where I interviewed him about his lifestyle philosophies and commitment to human and planetary consciousness.

Over the years, while cocreating the school and its professional certification program with my partner Joshua Rosenthal, Peter was a consistent friend and ally of our efforts. In fact, I still have a colorful piece of signed MAX art hanging in my New York apartment, with the tagline "Peace by the Year 2000." More than twenty-five years later, Peter and I are still connected. And the school—today known as the Institute for Integrative Nutrition—is the world's largest nutrition school, with more than 75,000 people now certified as "health coaches," and with an online certification program offered in more than 130 countries around the world. The seeds planted years ago have now manifested into a bountiful and magnificent harvest.

At twenty years old (the same year I met Peter Max), I found a mentor figure in the late Horst Rechelbacher, the brilliant founder and CEO of AVEDA. Surya had introduced me to AVEDA and its philosophy of drawing from plant wisdom to revolutionize hair and body care products. This was at a time when functional beauty products were an absolute bath of chemicals, and when nature and mainstream beauty were at complete odds; AVEDA was breaking major ground. When I met Horst at a (lightly attended) environmental conference, I again experienced the kind of instant connection that had drawn me so fiercely to Surya and Peter.

Quickly, Horst became a guiding light in my life. He was using business as a force for good, and it resonated deeply with me. I'd been attracted to the business world all my life, and I wanted my entrepreneurial instincts to coincide with my more "out there" interests that I had explored and developed with Surya. Horst was living proof that modalities such as Eastern thought, plant intelligence, and indigenous philosophy could actually form the foundation for a wildly successful company, allowing him to share radical wisdom with consumers on their own terms. AVEDA is and was aesthetically packaged in a way that drew people in. Horst realized that educating people about the environment starts with great design, a concept that is at the core of this book.

Horst was an entrepreneurial leader, an artist, and a revolutionary, and his vision drove me further toward my own. It was a meeting of the minds like I'd never experienced before. We understood each other—we effortlessly spoke each other's language and could seamlessly exchange ideas.

Around the same time that Horst decided to expand AVEDA outside of Minneapolis, I was in New York searching for a space for my school, which was gaining ground and had outgrown my apartment. Horst came to help me find the school's first home, and with his support and foresight I found the perfect location. Recognizing the interconnection of the lifestyle dots between healthy food and holistic body care, we opened AVEDA's first concept salon in New York—in my school.

Serendipitously, the web of Surya, Horst, and Peter created a powerful ripple effect as we inspired and encouraged one another and those around us. Surya, as a licensed hairdresser and talented chef, moved to New York and ran our school's AVEDA spa, as well as many of our organic/natural food, cooking, and beauty classes. Peter, Horst, and I shared numerous organic meals in the early years of New York's blossoming health food scene. Horst created AVEDA's first New York Institute, in which I was an environmental and health educator. And most "coincidentally" (I don't believe in coincidences), Horst's daughter Nicole designed one of the nation's first stylish organic clothing collections, Anatomy.

These bright lights around me—Horst, Peter, and Surya—acted as torches, further illuminating my individual path. As my personal beliefs and values converged with my professional world, I was able to have even greater clarity as to my true purpose. And I was drawn to other people who were undertaking the same work. When I was starting out, these people were few and far between, and we were living in our own universe. But I felt like we were planting seeds and cultivating them everywhere we went. And now, we're watching them grow. From a few free spirits, a new movement is under way, propelling a new era for humankind.

Living Life Under the Canopy

What became evident in my early years of embracing health and wellness, and its relationship to all living beings, is that we all reside together "under the canopy" of our planet's ecosystem. According to Native American philosophical traditions, the "canopy" is our ozone layer, protecting life and future generations. And the canopy also refers to the top layer of the rain forest, which produces much of the oxygen that human life needs to thrive.

As I deepened my knowledge of agricul-

What became evident in my early years of embracing health and wellness, and its relationship to all living beings, is that we all reside together "under the canopy" of our planet's ecosystem.

ture and the environment, I learned about the extensive relationships among the foods we eat, the animals with which we coexist, and exactly how our consumerism impacts the planet on which we live. I had an epiphany when I connected the dots between food and fiber, and learned that these ecosystems were truly interdependent. Hearing others refer to cotton as the world's "dirtiest crop," I became aware of the magnitude of cotton's effects on the environment, as one of the most heavily sprayed agricultural crops on earth. And I was surprised to discover that 60 percent of a cotton plant enters into our food stream. Given my familiarity with food and wellness, I knew how effective developing an organic movement could be for personal and environmental health.

At the same time I was unearthing all this information about conventional cotton products, a series of events transpired that I can only interpret as fate. In 1994, I was surprised to receive a call from the assistant of HRH Sarah Bint Khalid, Princess of Saudi Arabia. At the time I was fully immersed in the programs and workshops we offered at Gulliver's.

Princess Sarah and her sister-in-law Princess Hussa, who traveled to New York quite regularly, felt the buzz around Gulliver's, as Princess Sarah was interested in learning about the ways an eco-lifestyle could improve her fertility. She hadn't been able to get pregnant, although she had been trying for many years. Then somebody in her life suggested that if she changed her diet and lifestyle, it might help her to have a child. Her assistant searched for the best person to guide her, and ended up stumbling on Gulliver's. I started consulting with Princess Sarah, and ultimately her improved choices around diet and wellness resulted in the first of several healthy pregnancies.

Suddenly her cousins and sisters also reached out to me, curious about how they could use lifestyle changes to lose weight, improve their skin, and mitigate adverse health conditions. It was a little surreal—I became an overnight health guru to countless Saudi Arabian princesses. I had my network of natural food chefs cooking for them, bringing them fresh plant-based food, both domestically and in Saudi Arabia (Surya lived in Princess Hussa's palace for a year!). I was exporting organic foods as well as AVEDA and Jurlique beauty products to Saudi Arabia and other destinations in which they resided. I still to this day, more than two decades later, enjoy my friendship and consulting relationship with Princess Sarah, who now has three beautiful children.

Aside from guiding the princesses in the areas of health, we also had a fabulous time together shopping in New York. One day, we were shopping on Fifth Avenue, and Princess Sarah remarked, "You've turned us on to all these other products. You've changed our lifestyles. What about fashion?" At that point, the vague concept of organic and sustainable fashion had been marinating for some time, thanks to inspiration from Deja Shoes and my partnership with Anthony Rodale and the Rodale Institute—pioneers of the regenerative organic agricultural movement. But at that moment, everything fell into place, and a major lightbulb went off. I asked, "If I create styles made responsibly, will you buy them from me?" Their response was so enthusiastic, and within days I filed a trademark on "ECOfashion" and rolled my sleeves up, determined to fuse ecology with fashion. Shortly after, in 1996, I founded a direct-to-consumer sustainable lifestyle brand called Under the Canopy—the first of its kind.

Under the Canopy has always had a mission to give consumers what they seek in terms of style and comfort, without compromising environmental wellness or human rights. I have always been committed to breaking the stigma that you have to give up something to get social and environmental accountability—the worlds of style and substance are not mutually exclusive.

Under the Canopy was my first platform to revolutionize the fashion industry—through education, inspiration, collaboration, and innovation. Like Surya with wellness, Horst with beauty, and Peter with art, fashion became my vehicle to effect positive change. Although I didn't go to fashion school and never learned the technical language, I've enjoyed an intuitive sense of fashion based on a creative calling to connect style with soul.

When I started Under the Canopy, we were just a small mail-order catalog outsourcing many of our needs. We had only a handful of employees, and my sister and four sisters-in-law were the models. I always looked at the catalog as a storybook, where individual life choices of the early ECOrenaissance movement could converge. I wanted to seamlessly connect the dots among food, fashion, beauty, and business—we always supported this concept by using organic makeup and doing photo shoots at Whole Foods or local farmers' markets. The company had a mission of creating a holistic lifestyle, at a time when the concept of "lifestyle" was entirely new.

I had a blank canvas, and a vision of what I wanted to paint. But I had to "borrow" paintbrushes, and many people I approached didn't trust my ideas—they were (understandably) skeptical that anyone interested in fashion would ever care about the environment, and vice versa. But for every ten people who said no, there was always that one believer. With a meeting of minds and hearts, I partnered with these fellow dreamers to create something that hadn't quite been done before. And I was always certain that it was not "if" but "when" this concept would be embraced at a mainstream level.

Things really started coming together in 2003, when Horst and Walter Robb, the former co-CEO of Whole Foods, invited me to bring my ECOfashion concept to life at AVEDA and Whole Foods stores, respectively. For nearly two years, I built my team and worked hand in hand with Whole Foods to curate the ultimate store-in-store experience.

At the same time, I was meeting regularly with AVEDA executives to launch the first accessory collection in their stores and spas. From organic cosmetic bags, washcloths, and eye masks, to robes, slippers, and hair towels, our synergistic products and shared core values made our partnership effortless. Whole Foods and AVEDA allowed me to connect with the true beauty and delicious power of collaboration.

Until these launches in 2005, I was still struggling to keep Under the Canopy properly capitalized, with the high costs of catalog marketing and the growing pains inherent in a young business. But as the Under the Canopy brand expanded into every Whole Foods and AVEDA worldwide, these seals of endorsement were game-changing. Under the Canopy was on the map—and this was just the beginning.

I was thrilled and in awe as I suddenly found myself meeting with top executives of the biggest retailers in the country—Target, Macy's, Spiegel, Bed, Bath & Beyond, and others. Target decided to team with Under the Canopy to launch its very first organic fiber programs—bedding and kitchen textiles. In our partnership with Target, we successfully demonstrated that style, quality, color, price, and feel did not have to come at the expense of sustainability. They could coexist. And we found that our companies' individual messages were much stronger together than apart.

Since then, I've launched a film series called *Driving Fashion Forward with Amber Valletta* and cocreated the first sustainable fashion manufacturing company in the United States, called MetaWear. MetaWear is an innovative turnkey platform, which includes a forty-thousand-square-foot GOTS organic certified factory in Virginia—using solar energy to heat its water, seaweed for screen printing, and organic materials in its garments. The "Intel Inside" of ECOfashion, MetaWear is the world's first Cradle to Cradle–certified full-package apparel manufacturer.

Collaborating with organic food and beauty brands, environmental nonprofits, films, festivals, schools, and artists, as well as countless fashion and home brands and retailers, MetaWear resides at the intersection of style, culture, and sustainability. We're driving fashion forward by making ethical and earth-friendly production convenient for all our customers.

Along my life ride, I've also raised two amazing kids with the lifestyle I both embody and share with others. As my millennial children have come to see, their once "crazy" upbringing is now embraced by their peers—who relish connection, community, and purpose. What I love about having kids this age is I get to keep my finger on the pulse, and witness firsthand how cool it is to be conscious. They're living embodiments of all the progress that has been made in the past few decades. And they're proof of how fun and easy it is to live a clean, green, and mindful lifestyle if that's what you're used to (I never preached to them about being "healthy"—I was making broccoli chips and dairy-free pizza as if that was the norm). This journey is never-ending. There are so many layers of awareness, and I love continuing to learn and grow alongside my kids, as my daughter Jade shares in her note below:

Today I'm twenty-two years old, and I live with my mom in New York as she writes this book and shares her incredible story. Seeing tofu-burger alternatives, quinoa salads, almond milk at Starbucks, and kale on every menu at the restaurants I go to with my millennial friends is incredibly eye-opening, and I can see how far we've come within our mainstream society. Every time I step into our #greenmoregirls apartment, I don't feel at home just because I live here, rather I feel at home because I'm at peace. This is the place where I stare into our gigantic Buddha's eyes as I drink my green smoothie, listening to the most inspirational woman I know discussing with various humans how to cocreate a better world.

I developed an indescribable passion to "be the change I wish to see in the world" . . . the traits I was raised to value and embody—consciousness, health, kindness, imagination, and love—now shape my daily life. My endless gratitude for being an awakened and conscious young adult comes from my mom raising me with an awareness around what life really should be—traveling and seeing the world, experiencing every present moment, learning from mistakes instead of getting stuck, waking up with gratitude for the ability to breathe, a need to protect and communicate with the beautiful ecosystems, animals, and plants that surround us, truly pursuing my passions with love and human connection . . . suddenly my phone dying doesn't seem like THAT big of a deal.

Mom, thank you for teaching me wisdom, bringing me into the physical world, and loving me unconditionally.

Being a Spark of Light

It's such an exciting time to be part of this movement, feeling the collective, collaborative web expanding daily. A revolution does not occur overnight. It takes years of energy building, developing, and evolving. Like the Renaissance of fourteenth-century Europe, change is not brought on by just one masterpiece, or a singular thought-leader, or even one invention, book, speech, or philosophy. On the contrary, it represents a convergence of multiple ideas, leaders, and shifts. Like a snowball rolling downhill, change gains momentum and is ultimately unstoppable.

So the sparks that lit the bonfire within my heart took similar form, starting early, adding energy throughout my life experiences, eventually radiating to the outside world. In retrospect, my own personal eco-journey emulates the building of a rocket ship, with my life now resting on the launch pad, ready for takeoff. I invite you to step up—to bring forward your light, passion, talent, vision—and to join this monumental rebirth.

> I invite you to step up—to bring forward your light, passion, talent, vision—and to join this monumental rebirth.

I've never felt so excited and energized, now speaking on the "Seventeen Sustainable Development Goals" at the United Nations, business schools, and leadership symposiums on social entrepreneurship; fashion institutes on sustainable fashion; wellness summits on embracing an integrated ecolifestyle; major retailer conferences on plant-based innovation; and consumer events on living in a stylish, sexy, and sustainable world. I feel as if I'm part of a flame that's spreading like wildfire. And you can be part of this breathtaking blaze too. If we move in this direction of unity and symbiosis, we can fulfill our wildest dreams and effect positive change for all.

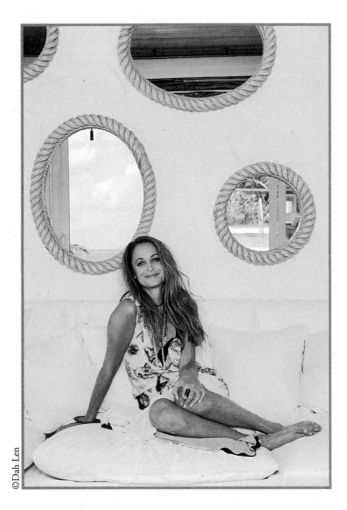
©Dah Len

Mirror, mirror: Everything is a reflection. An avid cat lover, I'm proudly wearing Stella McCartney sustainable fashion with a fabulous artistic cat print. Adorned with a sexy black onyx choker from Made in Earth, a soulful mother-of-pearl mala necklace—a gift from Horst for my November 11, 2011, wedding, which was also his seventieth birthday—and gorgeous black tourmaline rings from Joanne Stone, I feel completely at ease in my stylish eco-chic ensemble in this cabana at my favorite ECOrenaissance hotel, 1 Hotel South Beach, in Miami.

About the Book

Vision is the art of seeing things invisible.
—JONATHAN SWIFT

The name of the game is *yes, and.*

Both as an entrepreneur and a consumer, I believe that products and services should strive to give people a way to buy what they love and seek—*and* make a positive difference to human and planetary health, farmer and worker welfare, and future generations.

No compromise; it's not about giving anything up, it's about getting *more*. More value, more flavor, more beauty, more style, more health, more joy. If we can experience food that's delicious, satisfying, and nutritious; or fashion that's gorgeous and expressive; or beauty products that make us feel radiant from the inside out—*while at the same time* regenerating the health of the planet, that's the ultimate win. It really doesn't get better than that.

I'm a mainstream girl who wears mainstream clothes, eats at mainstream restaurants, and lives in New York City. I just try to make the best, most empowered choices possible every single day. Living this lifestyle, I've been able to change my life for the better *and* my friends' and family's lives around me. I'm immensely grateful to the people who have inspired and encouraged me on this path, so I hope to motivate and enliven everyone reading this book in a similar way. Together we can make this world a better place.

Welcome to the ECOrenaissance!

> No compromise; it's not about giving anything up, it's about getting *more*.

The Birth of a New Renaissance

More than ten years ago, I coined and trademarked the term "ECOrenaissance." I was inspired to name this book, and the movement it represents, after the all-out transformation of society that occurred in the European Renaissance from the fourteenth to the seventeenth century, ushering the Western world out of the Dark Ages and into the modern era. During this time, groundbreaking thinkers and leaders placed an emphasis on humanistic concepts such as intellectual identity, cultural movements, the arts, science, music, and an overall sense of self-realization. "Renaissance" is French for "rebirth," and millions of Europeans experienced this life-changing revival. Questions were pursued and answered, intellectual growth furthered, and hope was reinstilled in humanity.

Dutch historian Hendrik van Loon described it best when he stated, "The Renaissance was not a political or religious movement. It was a state of mind . . . their outlook upon life was changed. They began to wear different clothes, to speak a different language, to live different lives in different houses. They no longer concentrated all their thoughts and their efforts upon the blessed existence that awaited them in Heaven. They tried to establish their Paradise upon this planet, and, truth to tell, they succeeded in a remarkable degree."[1]

Of course, we have come a long way from the fourteenth century, yet in many ways we're on the tail end of another cultural Dark Ages. That notion may sound uncomfortable, and maybe even frightening. For many, it's disempowering to think of the current dire state of the world: we are in a time of crisis—ecologically, politically, personally. From climate change and natural disasters to drought, genetically modified foods, and chemicals in our beauty products, commerce has ignored the health of our planet, our bodies, and our children's futures for far too long. In fact, if everyone in the world consumed as much as Americans do, it would take five Earths to accommodate us all. As it is, the earth is warming exponentially, global sea levels are projected to rise as much as twenty-three inches by the end of the century (we're already witnessing a rapid increase in "natural disasters"), and species are dying out at the highest rate since the extinction of dinosaurs millions of years ago.

We're playing with fire, destroying ecosystems to the point where they're no longer able to continue their natural evolution. And in doing so, we're on the verge of driving our own extinction as well. These ecological crises have direct impacts; it's no longer possible to assume that the "external" doesn't affect us, as we all belong to one living, breathing organism. Human beings are part of nature, so when we harm the earth, we harm ourselves. Quite literally, our treatment of the earth circles back to us.

> Human beings are part of nature, so when we harm the earth, we harm ourselves.

Physically, what we put into the air, we take back into our bodies in the form of breath. Breathing in pollution can actually increase the risk of respiratory diseases: asthma, lung inflammation, allergies, and even cancer. Meanwhile, we're cutting ourselves off from our lifeline—oceans, trees, and other plants help to oxygenate the air, so the massive water pollution and deforestation across the globe are increasing carbon dioxide levels in the atmosphere, damaging the quality of the air we breathe—and the very systems we depend on. But we're beginning to realize a shift to the positive, to progressive growth, and to the light. We're on the brink of a rebirth—the worldwide process of renewing, rebuilding, regenerating, and rediscovering how to live in harmony with our planet and one another. Humankind is entering an ECO Era.

My vision in writing this book is to highlight the interconnectedness of human health and planetary health, and to help guide you on the path of healing your body and fostering a thriving environment, *with style*. In my decades as an ECOpreneur, I have witnessed so many people waking up and changing

> My vision in writing this book is to highlight the interconnectedness of human health and planetary health, and to help guide you on the path of healing your body and fostering a thriving environment, *with style*.

their lives to change the world. A fresh and magnified era of consciousness is finally dawning, one that's uplifting and accessible. People are asking questions, seeking purpose, and elevating their lives.

Knowledge Is Power

Although this movement is quickly gaining ground, the ECOrenaissance is still in its infancy, which comes with its fair share of confusion and misinformation. From personal experience, I have perceived that the biggest roadblock for most people in joining this movement is simply not knowing where to start.

In response to that, *ECOrenaissance* is dedicated to promoting further access to knowledge. This book is composed of personal insights, stories, and resources. I hope to help both foster your own personal journey and point you toward groundbreaking companies and innovators that are redefining good business. By shining a light on leaders of sustainability throughout the world, I'm going to activate your minds and hearts to new possibilities—to help you make a grand and positive impact, one exciting step at a time.

For many, the word "environmentalist" can sound daunting and full of sacrifices. And while it is true that adopting a sustainable, holistic, conscious lifestyle *will* change your life, you will find the shifts so elevating and fulfilling that you will no longer be able to imagine another mode of existence. In making more informed, healthier decisions and integrating conscious modifications into your buying habits, you will discover life-altering changes on every level.

This isn't really a book that will tell you to become an environmental activist—at least not in the traditional sense. This is a book dedicated to the understanding that embracing the ECOrenaissance green, chic lifestyle will make you feel empowered and enriched, instilling meaning at the core of who you are.

> In making more informed, healthier decisions and integrating conscious modifications into your buying habits, you will discover life-altering changes on every level.

A key mantra of the ECOrenaissance is "no compromise." I aim to revitalize the environmental movement, spotlighting ecological solutions for living both stylishly and symbiotically with the earth and our fellow human beings. The pages ahead will offer stimulating ways to make a green lifestyle sophisticated and innovative, showcasing cutting-edge design and ideas. I will guide you along my personal journey, showing how the world has truly begun to change for the better, and providing lifestyle practices and resources for fully engaging in the sustainable, conscious movement that is the ECOrenaissance. Gone are the days of boxy hemp T-shirts and gritty granola—welcome to a world where ecology is as elegant as red-carpet fashion.

This book also invites readers to adopt and adapt to this new age of conscious living through the engaging stories, tips, and guidance of today's innovators—the twenty-first-century "Michelangelos" of this new Renaissance, whom I call the "Illuminartists." The Illuminartists are the influencers, designers, ecowarriors, artists, and organic food, beauty, and clothing entrepreneurs who are creating revolutionary change in how we dress, shop, think, and live in a time of global ecological crisis. They're inspiring creativity and responsible innovation while tapping into deeper collective wisdom to align with current and future global needs.

At the end of each chapter, you'll find a collection of interviews from many of our modern-day Illuminartists, who are embracing the dawning of a new day of hope, preservation, and ecological living as both a celebration of style and an honest look at how we must move forward with limited resources in high demand.

> The Illuminartists are the influencers, designers, ecowarriors, artists, and organic food, beauty, and clothing entrepreneurs who are creating revolutionary change in how we dress, shop, think, and live in a time of global ecological crisis.

People from all walks of life are waking up, shaking off the blinders, and demanding change. This vast awakening has spread to big box stores, which were once the largest catalysts of many of our society's most dire problems. Internal champions pursuing solutions are syncing their values and actions, ultimately driving change at unprecedented rates.

Consumers are voting with their dollars, sending a strong message to corporations by prioritizing holistic health and wellness. And the message is being heard—retailers such as Whole Foods Market (now owned by Amazon) have grown into today's business role models, clearly showing that commercial success and environmental purpose are not mutually exclusive.

Mainstream retailers are hearing the message loud and clear. Costco is currently the largest US buyer of organic foods, promoting once costly products at lower prices. And Target is taking a leadership role, building long-term strategies and making game-changing commitments—making better products more affordable and accessible. We're starting to witness the ripple effect of the ECOrenaissance. Even huge corporations are quickly realizing that the alternative has become the norm, and if they don't accommodate the public outcries for more sustainable and ethical selections, they'll eventually be unable to compete with those businesses that are actually listening, and responding, to the changing times.

This is such an exciting time—with unlimited potential to shift the trajectory of the entire planet. Your choices can impact both your personal life and the harmony of the world around you. And as you begin to evolve and activate your consciousness, these shifts will just come so naturally and organically. As I see it, the change begins through creative collaboration, exciting innovation, riveting inspiration, and stimulating education in areas such as art, food, wellness, fashion, beauty, conscious business, and conscientious consumerism. This movement is about cocreating a stylish and sustainable life while driving new paradigms to effect positive change in the world.

Together we will dive into the depths of the ECOrenaissance to excite and ignite action in the six key spokes on the wheel of creative cultural change:

1. Art
2. Food
3. Wellness
4. Beauty
5. Fashion
6. Business

Ultimately these lifestyle areas are different points of activation. Initially you may be inspired by just one or two categories. Many people find that food and nutrition pique their interest before they develop their consciousness in other areas. But, as we will explore, these categories are all interconnected. One inevitably leads to the rest.

> You will learn to live in your highest fulfillment, nourishing the seeds planted within, while discovering space in the sun to flourish and grow.

Together we will engage and activate your existence in an interconnected lifestyle centered on the "we" versus the "me." And we will shine the light so bright for a better tomorrow that you'll begin to strip yourself of any walls of fear, despair, or hopelessness. You will learn to live in your highest fulfillment, nourishing the seeds planted within, while discovering space in the sun to flourish and grow. It's an amazing time to come alive—to welcome a rebirth and illuminate your life.

Before we start our collective journey, it's important to outline the most basic intentions, motivations, and principles—the ECOrenaissance Manifesto—that breathe life into this movement. These include questions you might start to ask yourself and others as you navigate the world around you. Shifting your perspective is the first step in any meaningful change, and as you reshape your paradigm, you will also usher in an exciting opportunity to choose a different type of living, where your decisions foster a universe of love and abundance.

ECOrenaissance Manifesto

What you think, you become. What you feel, you attract. What you imagine, you create.

—BUDDHA

ECOrenaissance principles to live by:
Be authentic; keep it real.
Follow your heart and trust your gut.
Always be mindful, kind, and open to new ideas.
Surround yourself with positive, passionate people.
Live the Golden Rule: treat others as you would want to be treated. And taking it one step further: treat the earth as you would want to be treated.
Cultivate self-care; laugh out loud.
See the glass as half full.
Be grateful.
Ask questions, read labels, think for yourself.
Seek no compromise when making choices.
Shift responses from "I can't" to "how do I?"
Don't give up.
Know that sexy, smart, and sustainable can coexist.
Support transparency and traceability.
Serve others, knowing your actions will ultimately serve you.
Be respectful to *all* living things—humans, plants, and animals.
Appreciate every moment and be present.
Build win-win relationships personally and professionally.
Add values to your definition of value.

Be part of the solution, not the problem.

Allow love to take different shapes and forms.

Remember that you can look good, feel good, *and* do good in the world.

Breathe deeply, be smart, and enjoy the journey.

ECOrenaissance questions to think about:

Do you wake up feeling excited and appreciative?

Are you learning something new every day?

Do you feel connected to plants, nature, and the environment?

Would you rub chemicals on your skin if you knew they were harmful?

Does the increase in natural disasters concern you?

Do you listen as much as you talk?

Have you found a creative outlet?

Do you stop to smell the roses?

Would you feed it to your baby?

Do you do what you say and say what you mean?

What does happiness mean to you?

Do you find the good or see the bad in situations?

How do you define community?

What is your relationship with animals?

Do you allow yourself to rest and reboot?

Do you have love in your life?

Do you consider how you affect others when making decisions?

What is your life's purpose?

Do you learn about the brands and products you're supporting?

What is your highest passion?

Are you having fun?

What do you think holds you back from manifesting your dreams?

How would you define your state of health and well-being?

What do you do to take care of yourself?

Do you trust your imagination?

How do you feel when you collaborate with others toward a common goal?

What kind of world do you wish for your children?

We're living in a time that's testing human integrity and even survival. How are you showing up?

Where are you showing up?

We've all heard the phrase "You are what you eat." Well, you also are . . .

What you wear.

Who you spend your time with.

What you put on your skin.

What you buy and support.

Where you choose to go.

What you focus on.

How you spend your time.

What you put in your household.

The thoughts you have.

The words you use.

How you treat the world around you.

Remember, every choice is part of you.

1

The Five Cs of the ECOrenaissance Movement

The secret of change is to focus all your energy not
on fighting the old but on building the new.
—SOCRATES

Manifesto in hand. Open heart. Welcoming mind. Thirsty soul. Now is the time. This is where the ECOrenaissance begins. Every movement has its fundamental principles. These five Cs are the elements of the ECOrenaissance; they are the earth, water, air, fire, and ether of this movement. Understanding these concepts is the backbone of rebirth.

Pillar 1: Creativity

Creativity is intelligence having fun.
—ALBERT EINSTEIN

As human beings, we are innately creative. We have the power to design a whole new way of thinking and an entirely new reality. Just think—we created everything we see around us. Just as we brought about the challenging conditions of today, we can generate the positive and lasting solutions of tomorrow.

Does this sound idealistic? It isn't, if we take it step-by-step, day by day. There's a learning curve—we have to experiment and explore. Think about it like learning to play an instrument. It comes in stages: at first it might be frustrating and difficult. After a bit of practice, it gets easier, but you still have to direct your focus, and you might slip up when you lose concentration. Once committed, it becomes intuitive. But it's never over—there's no perfection, and there are always more ways to deepen the craft if you so desire. Another thing about learning an instrument: if we're forced to do it, and we dread it, our efforts will likely flame out. We have to harness our creativity, our own unique mode of expression. We have to find a way *in*.

> If each of us steps into our full creative potential, we can collectively design a no compromise reality.

Learning the ropes of the ECOrenaissance works in much the same way. This green, conscious movement only works if people find their own voice and feel creatively fulfilled. While reading this book, you might find that one topic especially piques your interest and sparks your creativity. Maybe you'll find yourself experimenting with cooking, or making your own beauty products, or getting crafty with repurposing clothing. Maybe you'll even start your own conscious company. Find what speaks to you on that gut level—and have fun with it. If each of us steps into our full creative potential, we can collectively design a no compromise reality.

Pillar 2: Connection

Learn how to see. Realize that everything
is connected to everything else.
—LEONARDO DA VINCI

Nothing in nature stands alone; it's all interconnected. We're part of nature, and ultimately we suffer when we disconnect from our source. Just think of all the fundamental elements of life we embody. We share breath with plants. We depend on the light of the sun for basic vitamins. Water is the blood that runs through the veins of existence. We're in rhythm with the cycles of nature, with the moon and the tide. Everything in and on this planet feeds off each other, and we are a vital component of that. We're an extension of nature, as it communicates with us on a deep, intuitive level.

Reconnecting is the first step to flourishing and thriving. Every chapter of this book will reflect on this essential concept. In fact, in writing this book, it was sometimes difficult to figure out which information went in which chapter, because it's all linked. The lines start to blur between food and wellness, wellness and beauty, beauty and fashion, etc. You will most likely find that this is also true in your own life. If food, for example, is what initially activates your interest (I have found this to be true for many people), you will start by going deep into the green food movement. But you will eventually find that it leads you inward, outward, upward, and onward, connecting the dots between every modality for a holistically conscious lifestyle.

> We're an extension of nature, as it communicates with us on a deep, intuitive level. Reconnecting is the first step to flourishing and thriving.

Pillar 3: Collaboration

A dream you dream alone is only a dream. A dream you dream together is reality.
—JOHN LENNON

We're stronger together than we are apart. If we all bring our own unique strengths, perspectives, talents, and passions to the table, it's a potluck dinner bursting with color, flavor, and love.

Look around you, and you'll start to notice how many spaces are harnessing the power of the collective. For example, the new corporate architecture is all about open work spaces. This model is recognizing something fundamental in our nature. We strive to coexist and thrive in our ecosystems, sharing our space with similar beings. We're social creatures, and there's something innately rousing about being in a room with other humans, brainstorming ideas. A

> We feed off one another, prompting innovation, empowerment, and cocreation.

contagious, energetic exchange occurs. We feed off one another, prompting innovation, empowerment, and cocreation.

Pillar 4: Community

The golden way is to be friends with the world and
regard the whole human family as one.
—MAHATMA GANDHI

Whether it's local or global, micro or macro, at the end of the day, we are all one humanity. We all share the same, single and only home. We all live "under the canopy" of the ecosystem together, and we need to work together to protect it.

Community starts at the local level and builds beyond. Your community can be your neighborhood, your school, your office, your city, or simply your closest friends and family. Start at the micro level. How are your intimate communities shifting for the better? How can you contribute to that *today*?

Zooming out farther, we're living in the most connected age in all of humanity. The Internet brings us all into contact, so no matter where you live, you have access to a global community of dreamers and seekers.

We need the support and love of a community, and we need the wisdom of others to help guide us on our journey.

Finding and creating community are vital parts of this movement. We need the support and love of a community, and we need the wisdom of others to help guide us on our journey. We don't exist in a vacuum. Considering this, in each chapter we'll discuss how to both create and join communities in person, as well as connect to larger communities of movers and shakers online who are sharing their resources and insights through written, spoken, and visual mediums.

Pillar 5: Consciousness

Awareness of the inner body is consciousness remembering
its origin and returning to the Source.
—ECKHART TOLLE

Consciousness is, essentially, a state of being awake and aware, connected to our higher selves and to all that is. Consciousness is perhaps the most inspirational principle of the ECOrenaissance.

Consciousness is instinctual. It's our birthright. It's the "sixth sense," like fish swimming in schools or birds flying in perfect unity toward a common destination. They're just in the know. They've tuned in to something, to one another, to this unspoken language and bond. We're part of nature, and we, too, have that power of intuition. We've just spent the past several centuries disconnecting from it. But as we continue to evolve as a species, we will tap back into the natural wisdom that we all possess.

Consider the work of the HeartMath Institute, an amazing research organization that chose key places across the world to install sonar panels. The goal: regulating the heartbeat of consciousness. The way they're doing this is by using these panels as a doctor would use a monitor to determine a heartbeat. In these studies, the sonar panels act as the prongs attached to a patient's body. In the institute's studies, the wires connected to these machines are replaced by actual energy.[1]

When the HeartMath Institute monitors the energetic heartbeat in the "ether" (the realm that surrounds us), the results are truly remarkable. There are actual spikes and direct correlations between energy levels and major natural disasters and global catastrophes. In fact, one of the greatest spikes in history occurred during the events of 9/11. The results support that our collective consciousness created the enhanced energy levels. The additional energy was shaped by the immediate and sudden surges in the worldwide focus of our global compassion and humanity. That is just one of the many examples of how our consciousness is a thread that permeates all living beings.[2]

Consciousness is its own ecosystem, knowing inherently and intuitively how to spread and thrive. When we develop our own consciousness, we create an inevitable ripple effect. Can you sense this around you? Can you feel the movement starting to take root, to shift the common awareness? How has this manifested in your own life, your own level of mindfulness and desire for greater intention?

> Consciousness is its own ecosystem, knowing inherently and intuitively how to spread and thrive.

Humankind has experienced many massive revolutions throughout our time on this planet: agricultural, industrial, and technological. And now we're on the brink of a consciousness revolution. We're collectively waking up. And once we wake up, we can't go back to sleep.

Light Is the New Black

Thinking: the talking of the soul with itself.
—PLATO

Creativity, connection, collaboration, community, and consciousness—these are the DNA of the ECOrenaissance, representing a radically new way of thinking. At the end of the day, these ideas all interlink to form a sustainable, holistic, and fulfilling existence. These concepts are absolutely critical in my day-to-day life, both personally and professionally. They inform all that I do, by constantly reminding me to stay in resonance with my truth and to commit to living and working with purpose.

These five pillars serve as a road map to guide you toward this inspiring, empowering ECOrenaissance movement. Once you embrace these principles, you'll discover a more rewarding life—one where you feel connected, supported, sustained, and healthy. You'll live a life conducive to gratifying growth and filled with enriching opportunity as well as personal progress and self-actualization.

Are you ready for a shift? Are you ready to leave behind a world where you may feel stuck and lacking motivation or meaning and enter one that's lucid and on the cutting edge of abundance and elevated consciousness? Maybe you have started this journey by purchasing organic and hormone-free food; or you take public transportation or ride-share; perhaps you bring your own bags to the grocery store; or volunteer in soup kitchens or animal shelters. These are just a few examples of the small steps that add up to make a real difference and that are easy to implement in your own life. The shift can and will occur if we each play our part in the greater good of all.

In this book, we will address questions such as:

- How do we shift the paradigms of popular culture to be more in tune with the way nature intended us to be?
- How do we find purpose, meaning, and fulfillment in today's disconnected world in both our professional and personal lives?
- How do we reverse the ecological damage that has already been done—with no compromise?
- How do we make choices that regenerate rather than degenerate human and planetary health?

And most important, how do we choose to live a life that embodies the five Cs of the ECOrenaissance? To accomplish these goals, let's move forward together.

There are no problems, only solutions.

—JOHN LENNON

2

Life Is Art

A true work of art is but a shadow of the divine perfection.
—MICHELANGELO

Art is the fundamental language of the ECOrenaissance. Art is excitement, beauty, passion, and inspiration. Both creating and experiencing art can wake up our minds and our hearts, connecting us to the joy of being alive. It speaks to us on a level that can only be described as intuitive.

> Ecology absolutely relies on art. We protect the things we love. We want to conserve and sustain what we find beautiful, inspirational, and brilliant.

You may be thinking, *Yes, but how is this relevant to the ECOrenaissance? How does it have anything to do with protecting our planet?* Easy. Ecology absolutely relies on art. We protect the things we love. We want to conserve and sustain what we find beautiful, inspirational, and brilliant. We take action when we're moved, when something stirs us at a fundamental level. Nature often offers us the most picturesque examples of art forms. And frankly, I think that the stigma around environmentalism comes from the fact that some activists have separated ecology from the creative human spirit. It's come to be seen as a movement that's objectively good but ultimately boring, stifling, inconvenient, and lackluster.

ECOrenaissance artists are at the forefront of breaking that stigma, activating people and propelling positive change. They're creating innovative, immersive art and design experiences that draw on nature as a source of inspiration, using sustainable materials and infusing powerful messaging into their work. They don't limit themselves to traditional art forms or the usual art supplies. They push the envelope, define new modes of creativity, and are willing to use art as a commentary on life to motivate, inspire, and perpetuate much-needed change.

Transformative artists aren't always easy to define, as they're unique and rarely fall into any describable category, but their individuality and ability to think out of the box—and often to find solutions—are part of what makes them truly special. No matter the medium, ECOrenaissance artists tell stories, interacting with our hearts and souls—speaking to us on a gut level while similarly stimulating our deepest senses. Art can be absolutely empowering.

No matter the medium, ECOrenaissance artists tell stories, interacting with our hearts and souls—speaking to us on a gut level while similarly stimulating our deepest senses. Art can be absolutely empowering.

This chapter will guide you into experiencing ECOrenaissance art on all levels. Each of us can participate in this flourishing expressive movement, whether by supporting ECOrenaissance artists, becoming part of a community where art and sustainability fuse, or finding heightened creativity and passion in our own everyday lives.

ECOrenaissance Artists: A Force for Change

Artists both reflect and create culture. This is especially true for ECOrenaissance artists—their work is driven by a desire for change. Consider these examples:

- Jason Silva is a media artist and philosopher. He's the creator of a series of short documentaries called *Shots of Awe*, which he uses as a platform to tell stories and explore ideas about imagination, innovation, the human creative spirit, and the magnificence of the universe. One of my favorite Jason Silva quotes is, "We are the captains of Spaceship Earth . . . we have the capacity to overcome our limits." *The Atlantic* described him as the "Timothy Leary for the viral video age."[1] Check out his YouTube series Shots of Awe.

• I was blown away when I first encountered Chris Jordan, a Seattle-based artist whose brilliant works critique mass consumption. He creates enormous, colorful mosaics out of garbage that points to the destruction caused by mass consumerism. His passion lies in conservation and social commentary, and his work invites viewers to consider the consequences of the blind consumerism that produces such massive amounts of waste. Check out Chris's book *Running with the Numbers*.

• My friend Elora Hardy is the visionary founder of Ibuku, a sustainable architecture company that designs and constructs bamboo homes—including an entire green village—in Bali, where she grew up. Her company uses all-natural resources and works with the land, building homes that are both visually stunning and radically environment-friendly. I had the pleasure of visiting Ibuku last year and was completely mesmerized—it was the most beautiful architecture I'd ever witnessed. Check out her TED Talk "Building a Sustainable (Bamboo) Future."

• DJ Spooky, aka Paul Miller, is not your everyday DJ. He's a true ECOrenaissance artist, and his groundbreaking work has been featured everywhere from magazines to museums, clubs to stages, universities to conferences, and films to festivals. An accomplished composer with, according to *National Geographic*, "Multimedia Mixes to Save the Planet," Miller has composed powerful art that speaks to some of our greatest environmental concerns. *The Book of Ice* is his brilliant study and acoustic portrait of Antarctica and climate change, contemplating humanity's relationship with our natural world. His work lives at the intersection of music, video, animation, and science. "I don't see a piece of music as an end result; for me it's an ongoing process," said Miller in a *National Geographic* interview. "If you make it freely available, people with shared values can connect and create their own community. Imagination is our ultimate renewable resource. That's why I'm so optimistic that the past doesn't have to define our future."[2] For more on DJ Spooky, visit www.djspooky.com.

Experiencing ECOrenaissance Art

Art and culture are the essence of our humanity. They're everywhere you look, and come in many different shapes and sizes. From a very young age, we all have that creative drive, and we can all be active participants in the experience of art.

As we have progressed and evolved as a society, so have our art and art forms. Art is no longer a two-dimensional combination of media such as paint and canvas. It's progressive, noncompliant, without boundaries, and constantly reinventing itself to imitate something it once was. As we push the envelope, we find a dynamic and experiential version of art present across the board. Art has more meaning than ever before, acting as a social and political commentator, paradigm shifter, and conduit for our development of thought and progress. The examples are vast and endless. They're intentional, spectacular, surprising, and poignant in how they now imitate life. One in particular is what we see within festival culture, where tens of thousands of people come together to live art at every level.

> Art has more meaning than ever before, acting as a social and political commentator, paradigm shifter, and conduit for our development of thought and progress.

Take Burning Man, for example—one of the world's most extraordinary manifestations of human connection and collaboration. At first, the festival was a small, fringe event, but now it has crossed over into a mainstream mentality—with more than eighty *thousand* people coming together for this weeklong experience of art and expression. The energy of Burning Man transcends the festival itself, as well: Burning Man Arts gifts millions of dollars to more than one hundred art projects each year.

In 2004, Burning Man cofounder Larry Harvey wrote the Ten Principles, which not only reflect the ethos of the festival but also contain ideals that are applicable throughout our lives.[3] They are:

1. **Radical inclusion:** Anyone may be part of Burning Man. We welcome and respect the stranger. No prerequisites exist for participation in our community.
2. **Gifting:** Burning Man is devoted to acts of gift giving. The value of a gift

is unconditional. Gifting does not contemplate a return or an exchange for something of equal value.

3. **Decommodification:** To preserve the spirit of gifting, our community seeks to create social environments that are unmediated by commercial sponsorships, transactions, or advertising. We stand ready to protect our culture from such exploitation. We resist the substitution of consumption for participatory experience.

4. **Radical Self-reliance:** Burning Man encourages the individual to discover, exercise, and rely on his or her inner resources.

5. **Radical Self-expression:** Radical self-expression arises from the unique gifts of the individual. No one other than the individual or a collaborating group can determine its content. It's offered as a gift to others. In this spirit, the giver should respect the rights and liberties of the recipient.

6. **Communal effort:** Our community values creative cooperation and collaboration. We strive to produce, promote, and protect social networks, public spaces, works of art, and methods of communication that support such interaction.

7. **Civic responsibility:** We value civil society. Community members who organize events should assume responsibility for public welfare and endeavor to communicate civic responsibilities to participants. They must also assume responsibility for conducting events in accordance with local, state, and federal laws.

8. **Leaving no trace:** Our community respects the environment. We're committed to leaving no physical trace of our activities wherever we gather. We clean up after ourselves and endeavor, whenever possible, to leave such places in a better state than when we found them.

9. **Participation:** Our community is committed to a radically participatory ethic. We believe that transformative change, whether in the individual or in society, can occur only through the medium of deeply personal participation. We achieve being through doing. Everyone is invited to work. Everyone is invited to play. We make the world real through actions that open the heart.

10. **Immediacy:** Immediate experience is, in many ways, the most important touchstone of value in our culture. We seek to overcome barriers that stand

between us and a recognition of our inner selves, the reality of those around us, participation in society, and contact with a natural world exceeding human powers. No idea can substitute for this experience.

Sound familiar? The fact that these ideals parallel the five pillars of the ECOrenaissance so closely is no coincidence. By evolving and gaining wider and wider audiences, the popularity of Burning Man and the corresponding embrace of its values mirror the shift taking place in society. It's one example of the evolution and transformation of art, and how festival culture has exploded as individuals have craved collective community to feed their souls. Over the years, hundreds of thousands of people have come together to celebrate Burning Man by being *in* the art, the music, the sculpture, and the dance. They interject themselves as part of the masterpiece, designing art by following Cradle to Cradle principles, which state that what we take from the earth we must put back into it. Burning Man is living proof that people are starving for a way to connect—with nature, with themselves, and with each other. They spend their time at the festival listening to talented musicians, but also creating their own art, dance, and music. The synergy of their existence perpetuates a thoughtful execution of art, with the festival simply acting as the canvas for the creation.

And Burning Man's commitment to sustainability is unparalleled. Festivalgoers bring all their own food and drinks and take away everything they bring, including any trash. There's no electricity, except what is created using renewable sources. And it takes place in the middle of the desert, where blinding dust storms are almost routine. But this isn't an inconvenience—instead, it becomes part of the art itself. The mesmerizing installation and performance art at Burning Man doesn't stop at aesthetics—it's also innovative and resourceful. Artists are working *with* the environment instead of against it, and using the magnificence of nature as a source of inspiration.

We can look at Burning Man as a metaphor for the larger ecological movement. Who would think that four hours away from the closest city, in the middle of a windy desert, people could actually create a fully sustainable city of their own? It speaks to the power of the imagination when we combine it with the motivation. And think about what, exactly, motivates Burning Man participants. People flock to this festival for a variety of reasons, but it's very doubtful that anyone would travel to the middle of a desert to live without modern conveniences such as electricity, running water, and trash disposal, if that's all

Try This: Creating the Burning Man Experience

You can take the human out of the festival, but you can't take the festival out of the human. I think that Burning Man is a phenomenon that everyone should experience at least once in his or her life, if possible. But what about if you've never been, can't make it this year, or just got back and have the postfestival blues? How can we create our own Burning Man experience within our everyday lives and communities?

- **Connect with nature.** Find a way to immerse yourself in the beauty of the natural world every day. Simple daily actions could include tending to a potted plant or a small garden or taking a walk in a park. In the spirit of Burning Man, bike to work and your favorite destinations—and make sure you literally stop to smell the roses! On days with more free time, go for a hike or a longer walk somewhere more remote, where you can truly be still and connect with the beauty of the world around you. And this doesn't have to be limited to sunny, pleasant days. Just as the dust storms are integral and powerful parts of the Burning Man experience, let yourself be awed by the magnificence of nature wherever you are and whatever season surrounds you.

- **Form a community that gets it.** We feel supported when we're with other people who are growing, learning, and expanding. Our society at large can be confusing and chaotic, and while it's important to spread education outside of the proverbial choir, it's just as necessary to feel supported on your journey. And that way, sustainability efforts are entertaining and connective—if you feel isolated and exhausted instead of empowered, you may not fulfill your highest desires or meet your true potential.

- **Challenge yourself to limit resources—but make it fun.** The conditions of Burning Man make awareness effortless. People enjoy getting creative with resources because it's part of the overall experience. So, in the context of everyday life, turn conservation from a chore into a game. Each day, write down three things you could cut down on. Limiting—or eliminating—packaging, plastic (especially bottles, bags, and straws), paper, toilet paper, electricity, and food waste could make it onto your list. If you have a competitive spirit, expand the challenge to your friends. And if you have kids, make it a game, with prizes. (Tip: Bea Johnson's book *Zero Waste Home* is a fantastic resource for creative ways to conserve.)

there was to it. But when sustainability becomes part of the larger experience of creating art, expressing yourself without constraints, and forming deep, raw bonds with other humans, it's a no-brainer. Suddenly conservation has all these positive associations. It's no longer a dreaded "I should"; it becomes fused with pride at the very core of how we express ourselves.

The takeaway is that conservation won't work if it's joyless and austere.

People return from this experience with much more than they brought to it. They leave as artists themselves, cocreators who built something beautiful and tangible while residing in the desert. They practice sustainability in a co-op-like setting where they have to focus on conservation and cooperation to survive. The small city they create has no harmful impacts on the environment. It's a truly beautiful training and practice ground for our future needs.

The takeaway is that conservation won't work if it's joyless and austere. Ultimately, human beings want to preserve and protect the things we cherish, the parts of our existence where we find beauty and exuberance and creativity and love.

> I believe that art and artists have the power to shape society and that public art does more than beautify; it stimulates active dialogue and participation across cultures.
> **—Dorka Keehn**

Other Inspiring Art and/or Music Festivals to Check Out

Art Basel

Bonaroo

Cinema Verde: International Green Arts and Cinema Festival

Coachella

Grass Roots Festival of Music and Dance

Green Festival USA

Lightning in a Bottle

Lollapalooza
Sweet Life Festival
SXSW

The Digital Age of ECOrenaissance Art

If you can't make it to the immersive experience of a festival, art is all around us every day. Thanks to the Internet and social media, it's never been easier to experience—and to create—art. The Internet presents a vast global space where people from all backgrounds explore, expand, and create together.

Consider the example of Dang My Linh, a Vietnamese concept artist who uses digital technology to combine multiple portraits into one. She says, "I focus on observing people around me, the way light hits their face and changes color."[4] Then there is Alyn Spiller, a concept artist who specializes in environmental art. He garnered inspiration from the illustrious northern lights to create a recent masterpiece (www.alynspiller.com). Each of these artists utilizes the power of technology to create his or her art and then share it with the world, without ever stepping into a physical gallery.

In addition, their digital technology leaves no harmful impact on the environment, and leaves no carbon footprint, as some other art forms and their materials might. There is literally no waste. These artists transcend the canvas and follow their passion and love to create something different from what we've seen in the past.

But maybe the most exciting part of all this is the access new art forms can provide. There was a time when art was deemed highbrow or inaccessible. But now you can use the Internet or social media not to just access these transformative digital artists, but also to enjoy, learn, and take in the history and legacy of generations of art. And as technology forges ahead, we can only imagine the new mediums of creation we will eventually enjoy.

I'm a huge Internet appreciator. I think the dawn of the Internet, and of social media, has exponentially expanded the possibilities for human creativity and connection. Image-based platforms such as Instagram and Pinterest are proof of the powerful attraction of beautiful visuals—we're speaking the wordless language of art, designing and curating. And we're also being profoundly connected to other people, communities, and ideas through platforms such as blogs and podcasts. It's a shared, democratic space where anyone can start a photography or art blog, sell an album of original music, and even publish a book.

Artists tell stories. A stunning photograph of a rain forest, a powerful song with an urgent message—whatever the modality may be, art connects us to the core of the human spirit and reminds us of who we truly are. Art offers innovative forward thinking that perpetuates consciousness and awakens our curiosity. It leaves us with a series of "what ifs," which is the essence of continued evolution. Most of us are so disconnected from nature, how can we be moved by something we can't even see? Art draws us into the picture and allows us to witness what we can't experience firsthand.

Below I've listed podcasts, musicians, and films that I think embody ECOrenaissance art—and, of course, these are just the tip of the iceberg.

Listen Up: ECOrenaissance Podcasts

Personally, I'm new to the podcast craze, but I wish I had discovered them sooner. Most are free, and they're such an easy and fun way to tune in to fresh, innovative ideas and conversations.

- *Airplane Mode*: Traveling is the most wonderful way to connect with our global community; "experience the world through (and with) everyone else out there."
- *Take Out with Ashley and Robyn*: Grab takeout while you discover the inspirational, informational, and impactful stories of ECOrenaissance game changers.
- *How I Built This*: Artistic vision and creativity are at the core of these positively passionate entrepreneur and innovator narratives, journeys, and movements.
- *Lady Gang*: A raw, honest look at today's popular culture and how these power women unite in the name of transparency and love.
- *One Part Plant*: From Jessica Murnane, engaging and delicious if you're transitioning to a healthier diet and lifestyle; recipes and more.
- *Ritual*: A culturally connected podcast about "doing what's 'rite': how humans make patterns of meaning in a maddening world." Tune in, turn on.
- *The Pitch*: If you like *Shark Tank*, here's a softer, more thoughtful version to bring your ideas to life. Synchronicity and discoveries abound.

> I totally believe that the individual has the power to effect change in our global universe. In the instant information age with social media, our voices are heard and positive messaging can get through.
>
> —**Debbie Levin**

Tune In to These ECOrenaissance Songwriters, Musicians, and Bands

For these artists, green is a no-brainer. Not only are many of their songs infused with powerful messaging, these artists are also leveraging their platforms to create awareness in a number of ways. Many are vegans and vegetarians, and have started environmental foundations, greened their tours, and use organic cotton T-shirts. All of them have a deep connection to being conscious human beings.

- *Barenaked Ladies*: Have greened their tours with organic food, material repurposing, recycling, and waste reduction while driving global warming awareness at their "Barenaked Planet" ecovillages.
- *Björk*: Iceland's most famous environmental activist; her efforts to protect her homeland and the earth while inspiring others (such as Madonna to make her *Ray of Light* album) make her an unparalleled ecowarrior; check out her album *Biophilia*.
- *Bruno Mars*: A strong supporter of the Rainforest Foundation and his sister's organization M.A.M.A. Earth, encouraging the use of organic and eco-friendly goods and services while celebrating the arts.
- *Coldplay*: From the Global Citizen Festivals to their work with local governments and green groups, these guys take feeding the hungry and protecting our planet seriously.
- *Dave Matthews*: Using biodiesel, carbon offsetting and ecomerchandise for his tours, Dave's one of the most authentic environmental champions in the music industry.
- *Jack Johnson*: One of my faves with a deep commitment to the earth on every level; he even started a foundation in Hawaii to support environmental ed-

ucation in schools and requires all his distributors and producers to use eco-friendly practices, understanding that we're "better when we're together."

- *Jason Mraz*: Truly embodies the ultimate ECOrenaissance artist, from embracing a healthy lifestyle of organic food and clothing (he even has his own organic garden and eco-friendly T-shirt line) to greening his tours, practicing yoga, and sharing his dreams for a better world through his Jason Mraz Foundation, which helps sustain environmental protection programs. Love him.

- *John Legend*: A real leader, he launched the Show Me Campaign for clean water and agriculture; has greened his tours, invested in wind farms, and advocates for sustainable energy.

- *Justin Timberlake*: Honored at a recent Environmental Media Awards celebration for opening his own eco-friendly golf course—the first GEO-certified course in America—as well as driving hybrid cars and ensuring that his tours are carbon neutral.

- *KT Tunstall*: Dedicated to having her tours be completely carbon neutral; walks her talk in her environmentally friendly home, sweet home.

- *Maroon 5*: Helped develop the Green Music Project; avid supporters of solar energy.

- *Michael Franti*: A committed yogi, brilliant lead vocalist of Spearhead, and member of my natural products industry tribe, this man is as good as you get in fighting social injustice and championing environmental issues.

- *Moby*: Best known for his avid animal rights activism, this amazing vegan star is a true role model of human and planetary wellness; he created the moby gratis.com site to give music rights to other artists in exchange for royalties donated to the Humane Society.

- *Paul McCartney*: Passionate vegetarian and advocate of PETA, this conscious Beatle even helped create "Meatless Mondays."

- *Pearl Jam*: Big supporters of driving climate change awareness, renewable energy, and sustainability; check out their Ten Club.

- *Pharrell Williams*: Happy and eco, proudly creating Cradle to Cradle bionic yarns from ocean pollution with Parley for the Oceans and their Vortex Project (used by the likes of G-Star, the Gap, and Topshop).

- *Pink*: Lives a healthy, conscious vegan lifestyle and has spoken out against sheep cruelty in the wool industry and protecting animals worldwide.
- *Radiohead*: From vegan living to sustainable backpack collaborations, these guys are on it for the planet and encourage their fans to reduce carbon footprints by taking public transportation and eliminating plastic.
- *Sheryl Crow*: From biodegradable and compostable catering to reusable water bottles and her partnerships with numerous environmental organizations such as stopglobalwarming.org, she's working to live "off the grid" in every stage of her life.
- *Sting*: Founder of the Rainforest Foundation with his amazing wife, Trudie. An organic living and yoga aficionado, Sting is the original awakened artist, inspiring countless others in his industry to take action.
- *U2*: In the name of love, Bono is a true eco-rock star, from his fair trade clothing line EDUN to his work with Greenpeace, RED, UNICEF, Amnesty International, and beyond.
- *Willie Nelson*: From organic cotton tees to the founding of Farm Aid to his own brand of biofuel, BioWillie, he's the real eco-deal.

Earth Day Every Day: An ECO-Shout-Out for Beyoncé

April 22 is known as Earth Day, a day we commit to small (or big) acts of kindness to Mother Earth. Coordinated by the nonprofit Earth Day Network, it is said to be "the largest secular holiday in the world, celebrated by more than a billion people every year." That's an amazing fact. But what if we could celebrate Earth Day every day? Beyoncé lists six small everyday eco-changes that could result in a massive difference. Here's her list, and learn more about her other eco-causes at #beygood:[5]

1. Recycle your glass.
2. Recycle old cell phones.
3. Enroll in paperless billing.
4. Use cotton swabs with paper spindles.
5. Take public transit.
6. Go meatless on Mondays.

> If there's a goal, or indeed someplace to arrive at, let it simply be—living consciously. With that comes creativity and connection, two key ingredients of healthy relationships.
> —**Mikki Willis**

ECOrenaissance Films

Today everyone has access to Netflix, Hulu, Amazon, iTunes, etc. Take advantage of these platforms to watch some of these powerful social and environmental documentaries and narrative films. Some of my favorites include:

An Inconvenient Truth
An Inconvenient Sequel: Truth to Power
Avatar
Before the Flood
Chasing Coral
Chasing Ice
Cowspiracy
Earthlings
Food Inc.
Forks Over Knives
Gasland
GMO OMG
Home
Kiss the Ground
Okja
Racing Extinction
River Blue
Seaspiracy
Tapped
The Cove

The True Cost
The 11th Hour
Vegucated
What the Health

I love making films, which is very collaborative, and I love
engaging our amazing community in deep questions about
what it means to be human and how to create a better society.
—**Tiffany Shlain**

Try This: How Do You Become Part of the New Artistic Vision?

- Close your eyes, breathe deeply, and let visions enter your head.
- What is that one thing you've always wanted to do? Take a photography class? Study painting? Learn how to cook? Discover your inner artist and then begin to actively explore it. This is also an opportunity to be mindful and think about selecting human- and earth-friendly materials and ingredients—free of harmful toxins.
- What do you see yourself doing? Attending Burning Man, SXSW, or another festival? Listening to TED Talks? Diving into the independent film scene or discovering local musicians?
- Let yourself play with whatever higher thoughts or desires come to mind as you continue to breathe.
- When you're ready, open your eyes and feel free to write what you saw and felt in a journal, or perhaps in a letter to yourself—inviting yourself to bring your vision to fruition.

Living ECOrenaissance Art

Change comes from a place of inspiration and passion—never from a place of obligation. Imagine if everyone were channeling passion all the time—we would be living in an entirely different world. The ECOrenaissance is all about being empowered to turn our ideas into a radiant reality. We all want to thrive, just like nature when left alone. Getting into our groove, engaging with ideas and projects that speak to us, is at the core of this movement.

> The ECOrenaissance is all about being empowered to turn our ideas into a radiant reality.

Maybe you've heard of "flow state"—it's a creative state where we feel motivated and in resonance, where your body and mind are fully immersed and energized. When we're in the flow, we're getting in touch with the intuitive, gut wisdom that we all possess. Everything feels natural, almost like a sixth sense. You might not be able to explain your own flow, but you know it when it occurs. Time passes in the blink of an eye, and your deep focus seems to tune out all the surrounding noise. We're connecting both to our inner being and to something larger than ourselves. In my flow state, I feel like a little kid in a candy store—that feeling of awe, that I'm both living my dream and changing the world, is intoxicating. Add to that making my livelihood while loving my work, and I can't imagine anything better.

Try carving out a little bit of time each day and week to get into your flow. First, take some time to explore, and think about what activates your soul to help you channel your passion and creativity.

Try This: Join Me in Finding Your Flow

To help you find your flow, think about the following questions. Feel free to journal about them, exploring them as long as you need:

- When in your day, or your life, are you happiest or most content?
- What is the thing for which you wish you had more time?
- What is an activity you do for yourself and no one else?
- What are the actions in your life that are effortlessly rewarding?

Tips: ECOfy Your Creative Energy

1. **Choose a project or endeavor you love.** If you dread a task, you'll have a hard time losing yourself in it. A lot of people go through life in this state, not enjoying the people they're around or the work they do. Question this, and move toward an activity you genuinely love. This will probably involve stepping out of your comfort zone. Think about how you can infuse environmental messaging and/or materials into the endeavor.

2. **Live for the moment.** But remember that the meaning is in the doing itself. Flow is rarely planned, and often unexpected. Keep your eyes open and remain connected with all that occurs around you. Where in nature do you find your greatest bliss? The beach? The mountains? The forest? Integrate the sensation you feel in those moments with where you are now. This is a practice that we can incorporate into our daily lives, to stay connected to who we really are.

3. **Be willing to challenge yourself.** But don't choose a project so difficult that you feel intimidated by it. Finding the right balance of challenge and reward is key to letting go. The goal is to activate the mind, to engage in creative problem solving or artistic direction, not to overwhelm yourself. Imagine that you're a force of nature. Because you are.

4. **Find space and time that will allow you to surrender.** Finding the time is half the battle. First, you'll want to find a time that's quiet, so you can channel your full focus to truly drop in. That might be early morning, when you just wake, or early in the workday, when most people haven't arrived yet or are still getting their coffee and settling down. Some people get tired after lunch, so that might not be the best time to let go into your most natural state. Find a time when you have lots of energy and can concentrate.

5. **Clear away distractions.** This can mean turning off music (unless you find music that helps you focus), turning off phones, email, and social media notifications, and anything else that might pop up or make noise to interrupt your thoughts. Take some deep breaths, and calm the mind so that your space is clear—maybe even light some eco-friendly candles and incense. And then begin.

6. **Learn to focus on the task for as long as possible.** This takes practice. Start small. Commit to thirty minutes to an hour without looking at your phone,

dedicating your attention fully to your artistic endeavor. Gradually work your way up from there. When you find that the time is up, and you have been fully present and engaged in your creative groove, you have likely found flow. You can then work to extend this time. Remember that trees grow and flowers bloom effortlessly.

7. **Enjoy yourself.** Drop in and lose yourself—you'll find it exhilarating and invigorating. Note how your body feels when you allow yourself to just *be*. Flow is its own reward, so give yourself permission to focus on the present and not the outcome or result of your practice. Surrender. In other words, stay in the now. Be open to growth. Picture a soft wave brushing the shore. Yum.

8. **Keep practicing.** Each step will take some patience, from finding a quiet peak time for yourself, to clearing distractions, to balancing discipline and joy, to choosing the right task. Feel a sense of connection within and beyond, tapping into a vision of our beautiful planet in all its natural glory.

9. **Reap the rewards.** This is such a powerful practice. Once we realize that we can create anything we can imagine, the whole world is in our hands. Flow states generate infinite possibilities. An ECOrenaissance is imminent.

More than ever, art is about collaboration and creation in any form. Burning Man is one such example, but there are so many more. It's literally everywhere, and totally (thankfully) unavoidable. The amazing architecture of the high-rise you work in. The street-corner musician. The beautifully designed dinner plate. This is the maker culture, the do-it-yourself attitude of generations past, and we have come full circle to return to it. The abundance of technology available to us allows for access to tutorials and online experts, which support us in learning a myriad of things from the comfort of our own homes. This shift not only allows us further opportunity to be an artist in the nontraditional sense, but also to save money by creating on our own terms. And to choose what goes in and on our creations.

As it has been since the beginning of time, art is a way to communicate and express our innermost feelings. Like a bright light, art leads the way, permitting us to see beyond the moment. Art is the language of the ECOrenaissance. It is universal and understood by all. So turn up the volume of your inner voice—the one that craves creation so you too can become a channel for imaginative, inspired, eco-chic, and inventive expression. The

In an ECOrenaissance world, when everyone is connecting with their own creative power, there is endless potential. We can effect positive change together and have a ton of fun doing so.

beauty of art is its magnificence as a vehicle that can shape and inform our future. It's the understanding that we hold in our hands the power of ultimate creation. In an ECOrenaissance world, when everyone is connecting with their own creative power, there is endless potential. We can effect positive change together and have a ton of fun doing so.

The DNA of ECOrenaissance Art: No Compromise in Material or Meaning

- Sustainable, safe, and/or organic materials and methods leaving no harmful impacts.
- Driven by authentic passion and purpose, transcending the "canvas."
- Concern for social and/or environmental issues at the local and global levels.
- Designed via Cradle to Cradle principles (what we take from the earth, we must return to the earth), with a focus on minimizing waste and circular versus linear product life cycle models.
- Inclusive. No boundaries around race, gender, age, or ethnicity.
- True freedom of expression.
- Inherently multidimensional and conscientious.
- Channeled for healing and/or inspiring positive cultural change and/or renewed connections to the natural world within and around us.
- Innovative forward thinking: thought-provoking, lifting us up to higher levels of consciousness, and making a constructive contribution to humanity.

Illuminartist Interviews: *Art*

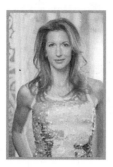

Alysia Reiner, Actress/Activist/Producer; *Orange Is the New Black,*
Better Things, Equity, Egg
www.alysiareiner.com

On- and offscreen, Alysia speaks "green lifestyle" fluently, and her
stunning home in Manhattan's Harlem neighborhood is a model of
eco-chic excellence and inspiration.

What is a personal ECOrenaissance tip you can share with readers?

Be kind! Be kind to the planet: commit to a travel mug. Be kind to your fellow humans: do something nice for a stranger every day.

What is your vision for the future of fashion, business, and/or entertainment?

My vision for all is that art, fashion, entertainment, and business all evolve to truly enlighten our community of humans. And that the five pillars of the ECOrenaissance are embraced and embodied by all!

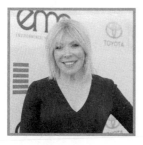

Debbie Levin, President of Environmental Media Association
www.green4ema.org

Debbie is a leading force behind greening Hollywood. EMA's
annual Green Carpet Awards is, in my book, the most stylish and
sustainable event of the year. Follow EMA's blog!

What is your vision for the future of fashion and entertainment?

We're in a very tumultuous world now on all levels. I totally believe that the individual has the power to effect change in our global universe. In the instant information age with social media, our voices are heard and positive messaging can get through. The entertainment world and our talent have the enviable position to be advocates for the issues they believe in. Using these voices for sustainability is more effective than ever in our history. And louder. As far as fashion, I see the fashion industry much like the food industry was in the early 2000s. Consumers are asking questions about what they're buying, what chemicals are in the fabrics, what chain of water use, labor, and materials is connected to the clothing they purchase, even where the clothes are made and how they're shipped. The answers are not comfortable in most cases. As we saw the massive increase in the organic industry for our food products, I hope to see that same account-ability for fashion.

What is a personal ECOrenaissance tip you can share with readers?

We're so fortunate that we have nontoxic and chemical-free products available for our home at competitive prices! Whether it's cleaning products, canned goods, fresh fruit and veggies from the farmers' market (or your own garden!), we can choose safe. Not only do these choices help keep your family away from seriously harmful elements in your home, but by supporting these companies, the products keep getting more and more affordable. In addition, we're keeping these chemicals out of our agriculture, which improves our soil, water, and air quality.

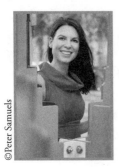

©Peter Samuels

Dorka Keehn, Art Consultant/Author of *Eco Amazons*
www.keehnonart.com

A curator, advocate, and all-around green goddess, Dorka is a true force of nature. Check out her book *Eco Amazons: 20 Women Who Are Transforming the World.*

What is a personal tip you can share with readers?

Eat less meat! According to an article in the *Huffington Post*, "If everyone went vege-tarian just for one day, the US would save a hundred billion gallons of water, enough to supply all the homes in New England for almost four months . . . and seventy million gal-lons of gas—enough to fuel all the cars of Canada and Mexico combined with plenty to spare."[6] Driving a Prius doesn't even approach the impact of eating less meat. According to the Environmental Defense Fund, "If every American skipped one meal of chicken per week and substituted vegetarian foods instead, the carbon dioxide savings would be the same as taking more than half a million cars off of US roads."[7] We'd actually be healthier with less of it, as too much meat plays a role in causing our three biggest killers: heart disease, cancer, and stroke.

What is your vision for the future of art?

I believe that art and artists have the power to shape society and that public art does more than beautify; it stimulates active dialogue and participation across cultures. Sites Unseen (sitesunseen.org), a nonprofit project that I founded, is a perfect example. Through a series of creative place-making initiatives, Sites Unseen is partnering with public, private, nonprofit, and community sectors to bring arts programming to underused alleys in San Francisco's Yerba Buena neighborhood in the form of permanent and temporary art installations and activations. The project will transform these neglected areas into a thriving cultural destination for diverse audiences by fostering social interaction, community pride, and economic opportunities while increasing residents' and visitors' safety and exposure to the arts.

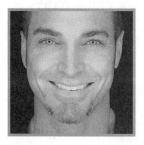

Mikki Willis, Founder of Elevate Films
www.elevatefilms.com

This elevated man has broken new ground with the most powerful movements for positive change. His verbal and visual guidance will move you on many levels. Follow Mikki on Facebook!

What is a personal ECOrenaissance tip you can share with readers?

If every big person made a serious commitment to loving and honoring every little person they encountered, our next generations would be empowered to break the cycle of bad habits and history repeating itself. If every child felt safe and free to fully bloom, from conception through their formative years, humanity would make an evolutionary leap.

How did you start your journey toward sustainability/social purpose?

Tragedy. The gift of tragedy was my catalyst. While in my midtwenties I watched my big brother slowly die of AIDS. Less than one month later my mother died of cancer. A few years later I was at the World Trade Center on September 11, 2001. After three days of digging for bodies and body parts, something happened to me. Witnessing the fragility of humanity and the material world had me snap to grid and get busy loving every minute of my life.

What is your vision for the future of media?

People-powered citizen media. That is, news that's not filtered through any corporate agenda. Of all the great historical quotes, the one that rings most true for me today is "the truth shall set us free." One of the most troubling details of this age is the explosion of fake news. Yet if you look closer you might see that this trend is causing us to activate and sharpen our innate ability to feel the difference between truth and lies. Whereas television has left us a bit numb and out of touch with our nature, social media is offering a forum to free our voices and awaken to the fact that everything we think, do, and say shapes the world we live in.

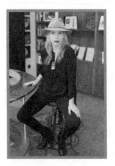

Tiffany Shlain, Award-Winning Filmmaker/Founder of the Webby Awards
www.letitripple.org

I've seen Tiffany grow into a true artiste and game changer. Check out her masterpiece film *Connected*!

Which of the pillars of the ECOrenaissance movement (collaboration, consciousness, community, creativity, connection) resonate most with you and why?

Collaboration. I love making films, which is very collaborative, and I love engaging our amazing community in deep questions about what it means to be human and how to create a better society.

What is your vision for the future of film?

The tools will continue to be more seamless—to be able to collaborate. Everyone now has a video camera in his or her hand. That is so powerful. Abraham Maslow once said, "If you have a hammer in your hand, everything looks like a nail." I would add, if you have a camera in your hand, everything tells a story.

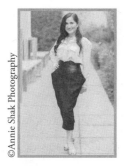

©Annie Shak Photography

Zem Joaquin, Founder of ECOfabulous and Near Future Summit
www.ecofabulous.com
www.nearfuturesummit.org

My original ECOfashionista sister, Zem is a passionate powerhouse with purpose. Join her Near Future Summit newsletter to be wowed!

What is your vision for the future of art and fashion?

My vision is a world where we're all #FashionPositive. Manufacturers follow Cradle to Cradle (www.c2ccertified.org) practices. Consumers understand what materials they're wearing, how they were made, where they came from, and who made them. In other words, a clean and transparent supply chain that's embraced.

What is a personal ECOrenaissance tip you can share with readers?

Never buy clothing made of mixed materials; 50 percent organic cotton combined with 50 percent recycled polyester sounds eco but is not, because though those are both very good options on their own, when you mix the two, the resulting garment is ultimately destined for the landfill. Cotton on its own can biodegrade and pure polyester can be recycled. Keep them separated!

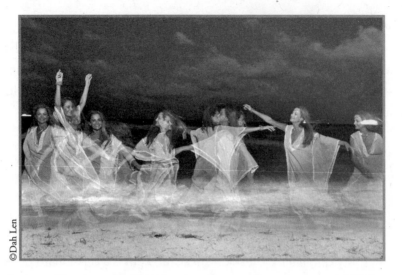

©Dah Len

In this photo, I'm in my favorite earth element, the ocean, at the quintessential ECOrenaissance hotel, 1 Hotel South Beach, in Miami. At the convergence of nature, art, fashion, and design, I'm literally dancing in the flow of this magnificent vintage Christian Dior dress.

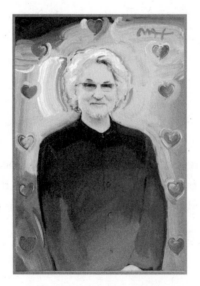

I felt so honored and grateful when I shared this image of Horst with Peter Max, who added his signature brilliance to this very special portrait—which he then hand delivered. Surrounded by eleven hearts, symbolizing Horst's birthday on November 11, this captivating painting embodies true ECOrenaissance art on every level: cocreation, exponential love, authenticity, community, connection, and consciousness. The ultimate Illuminartists, Horst and Peter are always in my heart, shining their bright lights on the world.

3

Evolved Epicure

Let food be thy medicine and medicine be thy food.
—HIPPOCRATES

Who doesn't love food? Food is a fundamental part of the human experience; it fuels our bodies, but more than that, it feeds our humanity—it's a centerpiece of social gatherings, holiday festivities, and cultural traditions. Food is how we connect and how we show love. It's so important not only to our health, but also to our identity, and can be a powerful vehicle for creating community and sharing culture. The ECOrenaissance in food is about celebrating, honoring, and protecting the beautiful nourishment that nature provides us.

> The ECOrenaissance in food is about celebrating, honoring, and protecting the beautiful nourishment that nature provides us.

But let's be honest—because it's so personal, food can be a touchy subject. There is so much conflicting information out there, it can be really confusing to try to navigate the world of food in a way that's both eco-conscious and in alignment with your personal needs and desires. But the ECOrenaissance in food is about no compromise, which means deliciousness at every level. It's about discovering a renewed, fulfilling relationship with food by getting in tune with what nurtures and invigorates both our bodies and our planet.

Many of the underlying principles of ECOrenaissance food define the idea of true harmony. The earth feeds us, and ultimately our own health is tied to the health of our environment. What's so encouraging about our current food movement is that people are waking up, asking questions, learning, and understanding that we're in a system of symbiosis with the earth. A reawakening is beginning, as so many of us are realizing there's nothing more gratifying than *good* food. We're turning toward a philosophy of food that uses the wisdom of nature as our guide while engaging innovation to propel us forward into a radically sustainable (and flavorful) future.

- Have you noticed the shift occurring in your own local area?
- Are you seeing more healthy options on the menus in your favorite restaurants? Or expanded organic sections in your supermarkets, mass merchants, and club stores?
- Have you started dabbling, trying new types of healthy food alternatives?
- Are you wondering about the source of your food, and how growing methods affect the quality of what you're putting into your body?
- Have you explored a plant-based lifestyle? Or wanted to try one but weren't sure where to start?

Whether you've been a proud health nut for years or are still a little skeptical about the whole kale smoothie thing, my intention is to guide you through some of the most exciting ways that food systems are changing for the better.

We'll touch on everything from large-scale shifts in the industry down to personal tips to engage with the food revolution in your own daily life and community. There is a powerful thread from soil to humanity, whereby healthy soil creates healthy food and healthy people, giving us the clarity to both survive and thrive. Let's explore the circular relationships that exist among our land, our food, our stores, our tables, and eventually our bodies.

> Better nutrition *better be delicious*—choose
> foods more often that delight your senses.
> **—Ashley Koff**

ECOrenaissance Food Philosophy

Food is a gift, to be loved and appreciated. The ECOrenaissance views food as a life source, as connected energy and nutrients that allow us to survive and ultimately thrive. We've all heard the phrase "you are what you eat." This phrase contains such a deep truth. What you eat becomes how you live, and the same is true the other way around—it's all interconnected. What we choose to eat can deplete our energy and harm our planet. Or it can uplift and heal.

It's positively transformational when we develop a relationship with our bodies, learning how to listen deeply and to hone a gentle, nourishing connection. The food revolution, the means of restoring our world, starts with each individual tapping into the needs of their own bodies while respecting our planet's resources. We eat to survive, but we sometimes do so in a mindless and habitual manner, losing sight of the ramifications of our choices—especially when they're based on convenience, conditioning, and cost.

> The food revolution, the means of restoring our world, starts with each individual tapping into the needs of their own bodies while respecting our planet's resources.

By changing the way we eat, we intuitively begin to crave foods that the earth has naturally provided and that are grown and prepared with love and consciousness. Many of us have been programmed from childhood to prioritize convenience and cost, losing sight of the gift that true whole foods offer. But food should be adored and appreciated, no differently than any other relationship in our lives. In fact, we should feel extremely blessed when food is so delicious and nutritious that we are literally in awe of its taste, texture, and source of ingredients.

How do we develop this mind-set? Here are some keys to being part of this fabulous food movement:

- **Make informed choices.** Knowledge is easily the most powerful way to develop into a more thoughtful eater. Understand where your food comes from, and the origin of its ingredients. Being a smart consumer is being a smart eater. Breaking unsustainable habits can be fun, as you get to explore new foods and different variations of what you've grown to find familiar. In most cases there is a better and healthier version of something you regularly eat. It doesn't take a lot of work, and it can create a lasting, positive impact on both your health and society. This is especially important if you're feeding children. The habits they create at a young age will almost surely follow them for life. It's okay to indulge at times and even have a cheat meal, but educate yourself on foods you should avoid as well as those to which you should gravitate.

- **Pause, breathe, listen.** With an overwhelming amount of options to choose from, it's easy to tune out, treating food as a mindless habit. And that's typically why people eat so much heavily processed, packaged food—it's there, it's cheap, it's convenient. But slow down for a second. When you're purchasing or preparing food, do a quick check-in with what your body is actually craving. Simply taking a moment to tune in to your body and asking it what it needs can make a huge difference in how you relate to what you ultimately choose.

- **Don't deprive yourself.** Sometimes, what our bodies are telling us we need isn't exactly what we think of as healthy. I've found that the absolute key to sustaining a holistic, conscious lifestyle is hearing *all* my body's needs. There's always a way to take a craving into account while still making smart, sustainable choices. For example: two of my favorite salty, crunchy go-to snacks are popcorn and chips with salsa and hummus. Stove-popped organic popcorn is great because it reduces packaging and spares you the suspicious chemicals in microwave popcorn. For chips, salsa, and hummus, buy organic, non-GMO brands with the simplest, most natural ingredients. My favorite combo is Late

July Snacks' Chia & Quinoa chips with Muir Glen organic salsa and Cedar's organic garlic hummus. If you have a few extra minutes on your hands, making your own salsa and hummus is easy, tasty, and filling, and also cuts back on packaging waste. Which brings me to my next point . . .

- **Cook it yourself.** Whenever possible, making your own meals—and your own versions of your favorite snacks—is a great way to connect to the food you're eating, and it's almost guaranteed to be healthier and more sustainable. Plus, food always tastes better when you make it yourself. A favorite of mine is cutting my favorite vegetables (such as broccoli, kale, cauliflower, brussels sprouts, or green beans), mixing with some minced garlic or ginger and olive oil (organic ingredients, of course), and tossing them all together. Bake . . . and forty minutes later or so, you have tasty, satisfying homemade veggie chips.

- **Joy and gratitude.** Seriously. This one is huge. Sustainability depends on enjoyment—new habits will only last if we take pleasure in them. It all comes down to bringing love back into our relationship with what we eat, and having true appreciation for the source of our food and its relationship to our environment. While I was in college, my dear friend and early mentor Surya helped me to realize the importance of eating mindfully and practicing gratitude. Before each carefully prepared homemade meal, Surya and I would hold hands and vocalize our thanks for the food we were about to eat. These lifestyle shifts were so powerful, helping me develop a deep connection with food and where it came from.

- **Eat seasonally.** Not necessarily 100 percent of the time. But when possible, eating seasonally (and ideally locally as well) is an amazing way to connect to the environment. In America, we're so used to having every dish and every flavor at our fingertips all year round, but that's not a natural condition. While very convenient, this system creates a strain on the environment, and I believe that it can contribute to a state of internal imbalance as well. If you're interested in this concept, traditional conscious food philosophies such as macrobiotics and Ayurveda give us road maps for eating in harmony with the seasons. (Tip: Kristina Turner's *The Self-Healing Cookbook* is a much-loved resource that I have read cover to cover many times.)

An ECOrenaissance understanding of food connects the well-being of our bodies to the health of our environment at every level. Arguably the most tangible example of this relationship is agriculture, so let's look at some of the current ways food is being grown.

Shop smart. The world is at our fingertips—use the Internet to find out what ingredients and materials the products you consume are made of. If you can't find a compassionate choice for the products you want to purchase, demand one.
—**Chloe Cascarelli**

From the Ground Up: Regenerative and Organic Agriculture

How often do you think about soil? Unless you're a farmer or have had substantial experience gardening or growing crops, it most likely doesn't cross your mind too often. Healthy soil is crucial to human and planetary vitality, but it often gets left in the dirt, so to speak. For decades, it's been depleted by conventional farming, diminishing its natural nutrients. But despite that, soil health isn't exactly a hot topic, even within the health world.

> We have to cultivate the understanding that true health starts, quite literally, from the ground up. Soil is the foundation of our food, so strong soil is directly linked to healthy humans and a thriving planet.

We have to cultivate the understanding that true health starts, quite literally, from the ground up. Soil is the foundation of our food, so strong soil is directly linked to healthy humans and a thriving planet. Let's look at the basics. What does healthy soil involve? And how is the current rebirth in agriculture renewing this vital source? And finally, how can we seek out and support these efforts to ensure not just a sustainable but also a regenerative future?

Healthy soil is critical for healthy food. Here are three key ingredients for healthy soil:

- **Balance:** Density to insulate and allow roots to soak in water and nutrients, with lightness to drain water effectively.
- **Biodiversity:** A handful of good soil contains more microbes (in the form of bacteria, fungi, and actinomycetes) than there are humans on earth.
- **Nontoxicity:** Healthy soil should be free of toxins (such as herbicide residues, allelopathic substances, and acids). Soil is sensitive to pollution from industrial runoff, which can be transported through water and weather from other nearby farms.

When our personal and/or professional relationships degenerate, what do we do? When important to us, do we work to rebuild them? Think about our soil in this context. Industrial agriculture is degenerative, destroying and depleting vital biodiversity and ecosystems, and perpetuating imbalance and toxicity. Yet we depend on soil for countless reasons. It's the mother that feeds us. It's the skin that protects us. It's the respirator that ensures human survival. In essence, soil needs to be carefully tended to and nourished so that it can retain its natural state of balance. But conventional food systems disregard the importance of thriving soil, and have thrown the foundations of our food, and our beings, way out of whack.

When soil is healthy, it's self-sustaining, and can protect itself from the elements (including adverse weather changes such as droughts). But when it's depleted and filled with toxins, it becomes weak. To imagine the effects of conventional methods of agriculture, think of your own body. Imagine getting no sleep, constantly drinking and partying, eating tons of junk food, and not exercising. You're more likely to get sick because you're lowering your resistance and weakening your immune system. But when you take care of yourself, work out, eat the right food, and live in tune with your body's needs, you're less likely to get sick because you're building your immune system, your home base. Your body is grounded and strong.

Now, compare this to soil. Soil is either going to be weakened or strengthened by virtue of the way we treat it. Food production processes have been streamlined to a fault, and it has come at the expense of vital soil and healthy food. Farms that once operated in tune with natural cycles have begun to produce one singular crop, year after year, on the same land—often referred to as "monocropping." This practice usually goes hand in hand with an intensive application of commercial fertilizers, heavy use of pesticides, a reliance on genetically engineered seed (genetically modified organisms—GMOs), rigorous irrigation, and heavily mechanized farming methods. Monocropping is a completely counterintuitive way to grow food. We are children of the earth, children of life, and we must respect nature, not work against it.

The GMO Debate

Originally, GMOs were engineered for herbicide tolerance; the idea was that we would be reducing the need for chemical agriculture. GMOs were intended to ward off pests, increase yields, better withstand the progressively unpredictable weather, or take root in depleted, nonindigenous soil that often is poorly suited to the crop. But instead, GMO seeds, used in conjunction with the complementary chemical cocktail of herbicides and pesticides, come at a high cost to both personal and environmental health.

The primary ingredient in the herbicide Roundup is called glyphosate, which is now being scientifically linked to cancer and autism. (As of 2017, the Office of Environmental Health Hazard Assessment (OEHHA) has even added glyphosate to California's Prop 65 list of chemicals known to cause cancer).[1] Because they go hand in hand, herbicide and glyphosate rates escalate with the use of GMOs, and studies have shown an uncanny correlation between increased pesticide use and the rise in cancer and autism rates.[2]

Did you know that every developed country in the world requires GMO labeling except for the United States? A majority of European countries have also implemented a national ban on the cultivation of GMO crops. And several other countries, including Algeria, Madagascar, Peru, Russia, and Venezuela, have entirely banned both the cultivation of *and* importation of GMO crops.[3]

We need to start reducing the use of GMOs. By virtue of inevitable drifts and runoffs, GMOs are creating concerns for sustainable forms of agriculture. The impact of GMOs reaches beyond the land in which they're planted, and, true to our pillar of interconnectivity, contaminate surrounding plant and animal life. We're a guinea pig generation, still learning about the long-term ramifications of GMO seeds and toxic sprays. Already, farmers are dealing with problematic superbugs and superweeds that have found their way into the agricultural system. These new living infestations have developed resistance and have been born as a result of nature's hunger to thrive, yet they present a whole new set of unknown challenges in ecosystems that have naturally evolved over time. The GMO debate continues to be a hot topic, with consumer demand for transparency driving a major push for labeling.

Advocates of GMOs have spent tens of millions of dollars fighting this groundswell, but we need to ask ourselves, if GMOs are as great as they're purported to be, why aren't the companies that use them leading the charge on labeling so that consumers can know when they're purchasing them?

If you're interested in the scientific data on GMOs, the Organic Center for Research and Promotion (www.organic-center.org) is a great resource, as is Max Goldberg of www.livingmaxwell.com, who shines his light on the importance of an organic lifestyle. Also, check out these organizations for additional information:

www.detoxproject.org
www.gmoevidence.com
www.gmofreeglobal.org
www.justlabelit.org
www.nongmoproject.org
www.sustainablepulse.com

Conventional, nonorganic agriculture is compromising our soil's health, because it's killing the good stuff with the bad stuff; the monocropping, GMOs, and chemicals are devastating the quality of our soil, our food, our environment, and our health. The good news is we can reverse these problems—organic and regenerative agriculture are critical solutions. In fact, it's imperative that we support a soil revolution to save us from global destruction. According to the Carbon Underground, "there is a 30 percent chance of human extinction within the next fifty years"[4] if we don't start taking regenerative agriculture extremely seriously. We need to draw carbon from the atmosphere into the soil to reverse climate change, or the runaway global warming we're now experiencing will threaten our very survival beyond repair. It's time that each of us plays a role and joins

> It's imperative that we support a soil revolution to save us from global destruction. According to the Carbon Underground, "there is a 30 percent chance of human extinction within the next fifty years" if we don't start taking regenerative agriculture extremely seriously.

the "Regeneration Generation." We are one collective ecosystem, and in the spirit of the founders of the Rodale Institute, who were the modern-day pioneers of the organic regenerative movement, we must focus on healthy soil for healthy food, healthy people, and a healthy future.

Restoring, Renewing

It's no coincidence that we're seeing a rise in health conditions such as cancer and autism. These are degenerative illnesses, manifestations of our disconnect with nature and destruction of our very home, Mother Earth. Many of us don't think twice about filling our refrigerators with food that's grown with chemicals that are meant to kill living creatures. We seem to have forgotten that we are living creatures, too. There is a profound intelligence in nature, yet our human hubris has divorced us from our ability to see and embrace the truth. It's time for a rebirth of who we really are. We're part of nature, no different from plants, animals, and other living creatures. Let's hug our home and give it love.

> The rise of the organic movement is really an awakening to getting back to where we once were, when we grew crops in harmony with natural conditions.

Most of us today have heard of organic agriculture. With certified organic methods, crops are rotated and no harmful pesticides are used, creating a greater diversity of nutrients to fortify the soil. The rise of the organic movement is really an awakening to getting back to where we once were, when we grew crops in harmony with natural conditions. The fact that organics have had a stigma of being excessive, complex, or luxurious speaks to how disconnected our society is—organic agriculture is simply a more intuitive and straightforward way to grow food.

But modern society has a tendency to overcomplicate the simplest things. Historically, organic food has had the reputation of being priced, packaged, and marketed in a way that was geared only toward a wealthy, privileged demographic. But there's no reason that has to be the case—organic makes more sense on so many levels (including financially). And as both consumers and businesses have awakened to the economic and ecological cases for organic products, they have become more accessible, and are even on their way to becoming the norm, not the alternative.

- **Millennials, who have surpassed baby boomers to become the largest generation in US history, are buying more organic products than any other generation.** And the millennial demand for ethical, healthy non-GMO products is growing constantly (in fact, millennials already account for more than 52 percent of organic shoppers).[5] With both Nielsen and *Consumer Reports* studies showing that more than 83 percent of American consumers are now eating organic food at least occasionally, organic food is the future of the food industry.[6] The paradigm shift is here, and this ECOrenaissance food movement will continue to grow exponentially.

- **The organic industry has grown at double-digit rates for nearly twenty consecutive years, as consumers demand to know the sources of their products.** As of the publication of this book, Costco, Target, and Walmart have surpassed Whole Foods as the largest sellers of organic products, and now even Amazon has joined the movement. These mass retailers are driving down the cost of these healthier and more sustainable options, allowing people to choose taste *and* value, not one or the other.

- **The demand is so high that huge corporations are recognizing shortages and lending money to organic farmers to increase production.** Costco is one such company—they have launched a program in which they lend growers money to purchase equipment and chemical-free land. In 2016, they gave the first loan to Andrew & Williamson Fresh Produce, an organic produce company based in San Diego. In exchange, Costco can source organic produce directly from A&W's farm. This is a major development, proving just how powerful consumer demand can be. And leading food brand Kashi (owned by Kellogg) has stepped up to help farmers in the expansion of organic agriculture by supporting the three-year transition of the land required for organic certification. In fact, in fewer than two years since the first full year of their program, Kashi witnessed a 663 percent increase in organic acreage commitments—from 860 acres to more than 5,700.

Organics in a Modern World

Five companies that are fusing consciousness with convenience:

- **Thrive Market** is bringing affordability and convenience to the organic industry by offering an online grocery shopping experience and delivery straight to your door—for prices that match or beat those of conventional food retailers. Their mission is to democratize organic products, and they live at the intersection of the digital and good food revolutions.

- **GreenChef** is an organic meal delivery service that operates throughout the United States and works with the best local farmers in every area. Their commitment to sustainability extends beyond organic ingredients, too—they offer vegan and vegetarian meals, and their packaging is made from 100 percent recycled cardboard.

- **Clif Bar** is a sneakily conscious company—their ingredients are almost entirely organic (more than 80 percent), and they source ingredients that are certified sustainable and ethically produced—Clif Bar products are available almost everywhere.

- **Elevation Burger** is a 100 percent organic fast-food chain (with great veggie burgers!) that has locations throughout the Northeast, as well as in Michigan, Texas, Illinois, and Florida. I even saw them located at a highway rest stop/ service station, where you'd typically find much lower-grade fast-food dining options.

- **Amy's Drive Thru** is America's first meat-free fast-food restaurant, spreading its plant-based organic fare across Northern California to start, and soon throughout the nation. No worries; if you're not lucky enough to have one nearby, you can always pick up a wide array of delicious Amy's Kitchen organic meals in the frozen-food section of your favorite grocery chain.

> It's imperative for the future of our species and the health of our planet that we change the way we produce, distribute, market, and consume food.
>
> —**Gunnar Lovelace**

Some of My Favorite Organic Beverage Brands

Bonterra organic wines
Califia Farms (coffee, plant-based milks and creamers)
Daily Greens
Forager
Guayaki
Kevita (Kombucha)
Numi Tea
Runa
Sambazon
Steaz
Suja Juice
Temple Turmeric (elixirs, probiotics)
Uncle Matt's (organic juices)

The powerful and rapidly growing movement for regenerative farming is a key solution to climate change: in its natural, balanced state, soil can capture carbon from the atmosphere. This crusade is all about protecting and rebuilding the soil, turning it into an organic sponge to address global warming—one of the world's most dire issues. Imagine a relationship in your life that has gone downhill—one that has degenerated over time. If you want it to be successful, it's not just about sustaining. It's about regenerating what was once positive and thriving. Now apply this mind-set to soil. We have done so much damage to modern-day soil and ecosystems that it is literally time for all hands on deck to fix what we've broken, while turning soil into our greatest ally against climate change. It's amazing how farming can be profoundly healing and revitalizing when it works in tandem with nature instead of against it.

What's the main difference between organic and regenerative agriculture? Regenerative agriculture, unfortunately, isn't always chemical-free at this stage. Its focus is on capturing carbon—a critical goal to offset global warming and the overabundance of carbon in our atmosphere. The main methods of regenerative agriculture include:

- **Composting, cover crops, and green manure:** Helps to diversify microbial populations in the soil, strengthening soil ecosystems.
- **No-till farming:** Tilling interferes with fungus communities that naturally occur in the soil and increases erosion and carbon loss. In contrast, no-till farming increases the quality of organic matter and nutrients in the soil, making soil significantly more fertile.[7]

Currently, organic doesn't necessarily mean regenerative, and regenerative doesn't necessarily mean organic. But the perfect organic system is also regenerative, and certain brands (such as Dr. Bronner's and Patagonia Provisions) subscribe to both. The best way to support regenerative agriculture today is to buy organic. These agricultural movements are bringing us back to where we came from, when food was something that we cared for and tended to and didn't take for granted. When food is grown with patience and love, you can taste and feel it. And of equal importance, our planet will thank you, too.

> The best way to support regenerative agriculture today is to buy organic.

More on Organic and Regenerative Agriculture

If you're interested in learning more about organic and regenerative methods of agriculture, these are great resources:

Kiss the Ground
The Rodale Institute
The Organic Center for Research and Education
Organic Consumers Association
Regeneration International
IFOAM Organics International
Demeter Biodynamic
Carbon Underground Project
Organic Trade Association

> When consumers learn the truth, they want to share this
> information with those around them, and thus become powerful
> teachers and activists in their homes, workplaces, and communities.
> —**Vani Hari**

Join the Movement: Kiss the Ground

1. **Learn.** There are endless amounts of resources available about soil, regenerative agriculture, ecological restoration, and the potential to work with nature to regenerate the planet.

2. **Compost.** What if every human were responsible for composting all the food they didn't use while eating or cooking? We'd have a lot more compost to boost soil fertility all over the world.

3. **Get involved locally.** Find out who in your community is gardening, farming, composting, building soil, and work with them. Can you bring resources to their projects, learn their local knowledge, and help share educational materials you've found?

4. **Connect with your food.** One of the simplest ways to regenerate the planet is for humans to live closer to their food. This could mean literally growing food at home or becoming a farmer, or only purchasing food for which you know the source. If you can see that your food is grown without chemicals, by supporting soil microbiology, you're supporting regenerative agriculture.

5. **Divest.** Do you know what your retirement account is invested in, what projects your bank supports, or how your money is managed? Transfer your investments to only ones that regenerate land and support ecosystem restoration.

6. **And it's not just food.** How was the cotton to make your T-shirt grown? How about the leather couch in your living room—did the leather hide come from a cow eating grass? Your cosmetics? Your kitchen table—was it FSC-certified, or did the wood come from the black market that's cutting down the Amazon rain forest? Everything we purchase and use in our daily lives has a connection to the land. Start to consider the way your purchases affect the land.[8]

Share your journey toward planetary regeneration and check out the Kiss the Ground film, book, and educational materials at www.kisstheground.com.

Plant-Based Revolution

I've encountered so many people who feel a sense of hopelessness about the current state of our planet. People tend to think, *I'm just one person—nothing I do will make a real difference.* I truly believe that every individual can have incredible power in many ways. But if you're looking for the most direct way to positively impact the environment, adopting a plant-based diet is possibly the single most effective thing you can do.

> If you're looking for the most direct way to positively impact the environment, adopting a plant-based diet is possibly the single most effective thing you can do.

The plant-based food movement isn't necessarily about going vegan overnight. It's about empowering and informing yourself, and implementing changes that resonate on every level. In the following pages, we'll dive into some of the most salient points regarding animal agriculture, the environment, and human health. Then we'll talk about how the plant-based movement is taking the food industry by storm.

Meat

Key Facts

- The meat industry in its current state is completely counterintuitive. Think about it—we're grazing over massive amounts of land to grow grains for animals that don't naturally eat grains. (Incidentally, human beings can thrive on cereal grain crops; if these crops were repurposed, we could end world hunger. But as it is, we're feeding half the grains we grow to livestock, while more than a billion people worldwide go starving each day.) We're using inconceivable amounts of resources to raise these animals: animal agriculture is responsible for 30 percent of the world's water use, 45 percent of land use, and a whopping 91 percent of Amazon rain forest destruction.[9]

- The meat industry is the leading cause of ocean dead zones, habitat destruction, and species extinction.

- It releases *more greenhouse gases than the entire transportation industry combined.*[10]

Why are we doing this? For what purpose? We say that we need animal products for essential nutrients such as protein, iron, and calcium. Supposing that's the case, are we destroying the planet for the sake of our own nutrition? And if animal products are so healthful, why, in the country whose meat and dairy consumption has skyrocketed, is the state of health in such shambles? Conventional American diets today are broken, which breeds dis-ease on every level.

Contrary to popular belief, even free-range, grass-fed meat is not sustainable. It's unquestionably more humane, but on an environmental level, it requires even more resources than grain-fed.

- It wouldn't be possible for every meat eater to switch to grass-fed and free-range; there is simply not enough land. Already, more than *half* of US land is dedicated to animal grazing. If everyone who consumes conventional meat made the switch, we would have to clear almost the entirety of North America.

- In addition, grass-fed livestock is much more resource-intensive. For example, grain-fed cows take fifteen months to be raised for slaughter, versus twenty-three months for grass-fed cows. That's an additional eight months of water and land used up, not to mention the accumulation of waste.

- All things considered, grass-fed, free-range meat can be as unsustainable as factory farming in terms of environmental impact, yet for those supporting animal welfare in farming and regenerative agriculture—following the practices of the Savory Institute—if one is supporting the consumption of meat, there is a case to be made for using livestock to improve soil and farming practices, ultimately to capture carbon from our atmosphere.

My Favorite Meat Substitute Brands
Beyond Meat
Dr. Praeger's
Gardein
Lightlife
Quorn
Tofurky

Eat plant-based protein rather than animal-based foods!
Animal agriculture is the leading cause of species extinction.
—**Kathy Freston**

Dairy

Key Facts

- Milk is the perfect food—for a baby cow. Every part of milk's chemical makeup is intended to help a calf grow into a huge, heavy, lethargic animal. Why would we stop drinking our own mothers' milk after infancy only to replace it with the milk of another species? More and more information is coming to light concerning the health and sustainability consequences of dairy. In fact, dairy is one of the most mucus-forming foods humans can consume, leading to a multitude of serious health conditions—from obesity to asthma to heart disease.

- Dairy used to be consumed and produced in very small amounts, to add light flavoring here and there. That mind-set was much more beneficial to human health and to the environment. But in the past century, dairy production has reached unnatural levels and has become an enormous environmental burden: one gallon of milk takes 1,000 gallons of water to produce; cows drink 45 billion gallons of water every day and eat 135 billion pounds of food. In com-

◗ Animal vs. Plant Proteins

Many people, including animal lovers and environmentalists, shy away from plant-based diets because they have internalized the myth that it's impossible to consume a balanced, fully nutritional diet without animal products. But this couldn't be further from the truth. In my experience, when eating a plant-based diet composed of mostly whole organic foods, optimal nutrition becomes deliciously effortless. (Check out the documentary *What the Health* at www.whatthehealthfilm.com. With Joaquin Phoenix as executive producer, this film is an eye-opener.)

The reality is, it's very unlikely that you'll ever be protein-deficient—it's basically unheard of if you're consuming enough calories. However, if you're considering trying out a plant-based lifestyle but are concerned about protein sources—or are plant-based already and could use a boost—here are seven complete plant proteins (and some tasty ways to enjoy them):

- **Quinoa:** Prepare it as a savory dish with veggies, or as a porridge with baked fruit and coconut milk.
- **Buckwheat:** Buckwheat soba noodles are absolutely delicious, hot or chilled. And if you're in the mood for something sweet, try buckwheat pancakes.
- **Hemp seeds:** Light, crunchy, and delightful on a salad, noodle dish, or grain bowl. Check out Manitoba Harvest's Hemp Hearts.
- **Chia seeds:** These gelatinous little seeds are great in smoothies and puddings.
- **Pumpkin seeds:** Toss these on top of a salad or avocado toast, or eat them by themselves as a snack.
- **Soy:** Soy products are so versatile, you can make almost anything. (Just make sure to always buy certified organic—conventional GMO soy is one of the most heavily sprayed crops in agriculture.) If you haven't already done so, try tempeh, my personal favorite of the soy protein family.
- **Spirulina:** Drink it in a smoothie or juice for a blast of plant-based energy.

If you're interested in learning more, One Green Planet's *The Ultimate Guide to Plant-Based Nutrition* is an incredibly comprehensive and thorough guide: http://www.onegreenplanet.org/natural-health/plant-based-vegan-nutrition-guide/.

parison, the whole human population drinks 5.2 billion gallons of water and eats 21 billion pounds of food per day.[11]

- According to the World Wildlife Fund (WWF), "Millions of farmers world-wide tend approximately 270 million dairy cows to produce milk. Milk production impacts the environment in various ways, and the scale of these impacts depends on the practices of the dairy farmers and feed growers. Dairy cows and their manure produce greenhouse gas emissions, which contribute to climate change. Poor handling of manure and fertilizers can degrade local water resources. And unsustainable dairy farming and feed production can lead to the loss of ecologically important areas, such as prairies, wetlands, and forests."[12]

Dairy Substitutes

Thankfully, there are endless "dairy-like" alternatives available to consumers. If you choose to eliminate dairy altogether, you're in luck, because now there is such a wide array of different kinds of tasty healthy nut and grain "milks," "cheeses," and "ice creams": coconut, almond, rice, cashew, macadamia, hemp, and pistachio. (It's generally best to avoid soy milk unless it's organic, since soy can be filled with GMOs.) For a nondairy

Did You Know?

John Robbins, son of the founder of Baskin-Robbins, found the conventional dairy industry so cruel and corrupt, and milk products and sugar so harmful to people's health, that he refused to take over the company that was to be his destined legacy. Once he started visiting the dairy farms from which Baskin-Robbins was sourcing their products, he was mortified by the treatment of the cows, began doing more research into the horrors of the food industry, and eventually wrote a book called *Diet for a New America*, which was a groundbreaking, hugely influential exposé in the early 1990s. Robbins literally turned down a fortune because he didn't believe in the food system that was being perpetuated by his own family's company. His book continues to enlighten people to this day.

consumer like me, I'm amazed by the delicious and fun alternatives available. Some of my favorite brands for plant-based dairy products include:

Califia
Chao Creamery
Daiya
Follow Your Heart
Hampton Creek
Heidi Ho
Kite Hill
Miyoko's Kitchen
Ripple

Seafood

Key Facts

- *National Geographic* states that if we don't reverse the ecosystem devastation caused by overfishing, we will have fishless oceans by 2048. Ninety percent of global fish stocks are overfished or fully fished.[13]

- And with our oceans contaminated with mercury, nuclear waste, PCBs, dioxins, and microfibers (plastic debris from textiles and other products that pollute the ocean and end up in our food), there are scary health impacts of eating seafood. Women are warned not to eat certain fish during pregnancy because they're sustaining a new life, but we're sustaining our own lives every day!

- According to the WWF: "Eighty-five percent of the world's marine stocks are either fully exploited or overfished, driving accelerated growth in the farmed seafood industry."[14]

The detrimental impact of overexploiting our marine wildlife has created an increasingly high demand for farmed seafood, also known as aquaculture. It's important to point out that this industry has its own ecological impact:

- Antibiotics and other chemicals used in aquaculture cause concern in terms of wider aquatic habitats and human consumption.
- Fish farms take huge amounts of space, both on land and in natural waterways and at sea.
- Excess food and fish waste from aquaculture increase levels of nutrients in the water and can lead to oxygen-deprived waters that stress aquatic life.[15]

Seafood Substitutes

Until now, the market for plant-based seafood products has been limited. But in 2018, my consulting agency BeyondBrands is launching a groundbreaking, flavor-forward brand of plant-based seafood—Good Catch (www.goodcatchfoods.com)—loaded with delicious, healthy, and innovative alternative ingredients such as GMO-free chickpeas, fava beans, peas, navy beans, soy, and lentil proteins.

The beauty of plant-based proteins is that they're able to mimic their animal counterparts in both taste and nutrient levels—and without harming living creatures, our vital ecosystems, or human health. Good Catch's fish-free tuna harnesses the nutritional powerhouse of algae oil (from algae that's farmed sustainably, in a contained environment), providing just as much protein, omega oils, and other essential nutrients as tuna itself—minus the mercury and pollution.

The plant-based revolution is about the realization that there is a

---

Whereas a vegetarian or vegan diet used to be seen as restrictive, now it has become one of the most interesting and diverse culinary experiences in the food world.

Try This: Recipes

When it comes to finding recipes to explore, there are thousands of websites, blogs, and apps to pick from, but here are a few standouts:

Alicia Silverstone's The Kind Life website
Clean Food Dirty Girl
Food Heaven
Food Monster App
Epicurious
Hooked
Oh She Glows
Vegetarian Times

whole world of fresh, colorful, delicious vegetarian and vegan fare that you may never have been exposed to. Whereas a vegetarian or vegan diet used to be seen as restrictive, now it has become one of the most interesting and diverse culinary experiences in the food world. Plant-based eating is all about abundance—making sustainability, regenerative practices, and consciousness delicious.

🐟 Try This: Plant-Based While Traveling

If you're still new to a veg-friendly lifestyle, traveling can seem like a roadblock to healthy, conscious living. Airports and train stations don't exactly have reputations as holistic health centers. And while you've probably found—or will find—that plant-based eating is incredibly affordable, intuitive, and enjoyable when you're in your kitchen or at your favorite local restaurant, traveling can throw a potential wrench into your routine.

However, in the past few years, I've been amazed to witness how much easier it's become, as so many people have been drawn to this movement. When I became a vegetarian at age sixteen, it was almost impossible. But now, plant-based eating seems to have spread almost everywhere. In fact, as I write this book, my daughter is traveling throughout Southeast Asia and is thrilled at how easy it has been for her to discover and dine at vegan restaurants. And for as long as I've been vegetarian, I have been thrilled by the growing networks and communities that have been built around this creative, empowering, and conscious lifestyle.

Here are some tips for maintaining your plant-based lifestyle away from home:

- **For airports, train stations, road trips, etc.:** Look for health-conscious chains such as SweetGreen, Veggie Grill, Cava Mezze, Lyfe Kitchen, Freshii, or CIBO. International restaurants such as Le Pain Quotidien, Au Bon Pain, Panera Bread, Pret A Manger, and Chipotle have expanded their plant-based menus, responding to a growing demand. Even pizza chains such as Domino's, MOD Pizza, Pieology, and Mellow Mushroom offer vegan options.

- **Once you've arrived:** If you're looking for a meal out on the town, happycow.com is one of my favorite resources for discovering the local herbivore scene. In addition, browsing vegan travel blogs is a great way to get the scoop on vegan and vegetarian restaurants wherever you go. Check out vegantravel.com, thenomadicvegan.com, and veganmiam.com.

Wicked Healthy Foods

Brothers Derek and Chad Sarno are world-leading plant-based chefs and the founders of Wicked Healthy Foods. Here are some fantastic Wicked Healthy tips to adopting a healthier diet. Pick up their wicked amazing cookbook and check the Sarno brothers out at wickedhealthyfood.com—"80 percent healthy, 20 percent wicked, 100 percent sexy."[16]

- **Shopping smarts are crucial.** Learn how to shop and fill your basket. Stay out of the middle aisles as much as you can; spend most of your time in bulk and produce.

- **Taking control of your health starts in the kitchen.** Being empowered when you open up that fridge and knowing how to create delicious dishes with what you have on hand come down to understanding foundational cooking techniques. Knowing the basics puts you in the driver's seat and makes cooking way more enjoyable.

- **Explore new foods.** Try to step out of your comfort zone with different ingredients. The plant world is vast with opportunities and options, it will blow you away with the variety, and there are endless options within the produce and bulk sections. With more than eight hundred varieties of beans, and hundreds of different fruits and vegetables, let ingredients help guide you in the kitchen with some creative and unique new flavors, textures, and dishes.

- **Educate yourself.** Knowledge is power, especially when it comes to getting inspired in the kitchen.

They also recommended some great blogs for the fellow plant-pusher:

AppleseedCuisine.com
Avantgardevegan.com
Hotforfoodblog.com
MinimalistBaker.com

Olivesfordinner.com
SimnettNutrition.com
Thugkitchen.com
VeganRicha.com
Veganyackattack.com
Wickedhealthyfood.com

Next, the Wicked Healthy brothers recommended that we grab those knives, load that fridge with plants, and dive into these killer cookbooks, which will be sure to crack the whip of motivation:

Crazy Sexy Kitchen
Crossroads Kitchen
Vegan Richa's Everyday Kitchen
Vegetarian Flavor Bible—the best reference book for flavor development
Wicked Healthy Cookbook

The kind of life you choose to lead is defined by the moral choices you make every single day—make choices you can be proud of.
—Leilani Munter

Food Documentaries to Watch

Rather sit back and watch a film? Here are some that will lift that veil and motivate change:

Cowspiracy
Forks over Knives
Game Changers (2018)
Hungry for Change
Okja

Plant Pure Nation
Vegucated
What the Health

Urban Agriculture

It's so exciting to watch the abundance of innovations in the way food is being grown, distributed, experienced, and enjoyed. Organic and regenerative agriculture and the plant-based movement are changing the world of food, but they're just the tip of the iceberg. There are countless other ways to join the food ECOrenaissance.

Currently we're witnessing people from the smallest towns to the most bustling cities coming together to connect with the foundations of food. The revolution in agriculture is all about coming full circle, meeting the wisdom of the past with the very real needs of a globalized, heavily populated world. People everywhere are realizing that we can't keep going with the same ideology that has created food shortages, immense waste, obesity, and the deterioration of health that has characterized the food industry for decades.

> The revolution in agriculture is all about coming full circle, meeting the wisdom of the past with the very real needs of a globalized, heavily populated world.

People are craving a renewed connection to the source of our food, and we're experiencing an absolute boom in urban agriculture, with urban vegetation walls, rooftop gardens, and community gardens cropping up everywhere, making it easy to "go green" even while dwelling in the heart of a big city.

- **Urban vegetation walls.** Also known as vertical gardens, ecowalls, or green walls, they're beautiful, living artworks that bring life to city structures while making the air cleaner and more breathable. They help reduce pollution and increase biodiversity—not to mention their effects on human psychological health. Exposure to nature enhances our peace and well-being. Studies have even shown that having plants in offices and other work environments improves worker productivity and attention and reduces stress.[17]

- **Rooftop gardens.** How can local get any better than when food is grown on your own roof? Rooftop gardens are gaining popularity as another way to ECOfy urban spaces. Like green walls, rooftop gardens help reduce air pollution and increase biodiversity. They also cool down a building, reducing the need for air-conditioning during warmer months. Rooftop gardens are linked to the popular Farm to Table and local food movements. They significantly reduce energy that gets accumulated in food shipping, and ensure access to fresh and seasonal foods. They also create a sense of community, and provide a slice of rural charm and comfort in the midst of city life.

- **Community gardens.** A "you plant it, you pick it" policy offers locals the opportunity to come together and build a beautiful garden filled with organic and pesticide-free fruits, veggies, and other produce. Not only do creative and collaborative projects such as these instill both a sense of connection with nature and a conscious feeling of positive camaraderie, they also help the community at large, as many urban gardens also donate several thousand servings of food to soup kitchens every year. These are cropping up nationwide, so if you're interested in connecting with your local community garden, you can find more information at communitygarden.org.

The positive impacts of urban agriculture are so clear that members of Congress are keeping up with this movement, instituting inspiring changes.

- **The Urban Agriculture Act of 2016:** This act supports urban farming initiatives and supplies grants for community gardens while increasing funding for municipal composting and incentivizing food waste reduction.

- **Future Organic Farmers Grant:** This is a program that educates young kids about organics and other food solutions. Programs like this one are crucial, as the average American farmer's age is fifty-eight years old, and approximately two-thirds of farmland will be changing hands in the next decade.

- **The National Young Farmers Coalition:** Currently it's discouragingly difficult for young people to get access to land grants. The National Young Farmers Coalition is one organization that aims to change that, supporting young people interested in farming at both the policy and practical levels. It provides funding and support throughout some of the initial challenges of the first few years (even supplying an exchange that helps college grads pay off student loans).

Don't Scrap It: Addressing Food Waste

The magnitude of the food waste crisis is astounding. We can't waste any more time not addressing this issue:

- In the United States, we're throwing out a whopping *40 percent* of our food; meanwhile, a billion people worldwide are going hungry.[18]
- Food worth $161 billion is uneaten at food retailers, restaurants, and homes—that amounts to $1,500 per capita per year.[19]
- An estimated 4 to 10 percent of food bought by restaurants is thrown out before it even reaches a table!

We have a national crisis, and we need a national solution. We need to take comprehensive steps to reduce food waste on farms, at food institutions, and in homes. For example, consumers are throwing away perfectly edible food based on expiration dates, so it's important to create education and awareness surrounding this. We're beginning to see action being taken at the policy level, in terms of tax benefits for food bank donations, and incentives for cafeterias to buy "ugly foods" (produce that may be bruised or off-color but is completely natural, nourishing, and nutritionally sound).

In fact, if we redirected just 15 percent of food waste, we could cut the number of food-insecure Americans in half.

Maine congresswoman Chellie Pingree has introduced two pieces of legislation to help combat this growing issue: the Food Recovery Act and the Food Date Labeling Act. She's working on diverting the amount of food that's unnecessarily discarded. In fact, if we redirected just 15 percent of food waste, we could cut the number of food-insecure Americans in half.

Both business and government are rallying behind the food waste reduction movement. Here are a few examples of businesses that are successfully addressing the food waste issue:

- **MOM's Organic Markets,** a forward-thinking grocery store chain experiencing positive growth and expansion, is leading the charge on eliminating food waste. For thirty years they have had an environmental coordinator who oversees food recovery, using ugly produce in cafés or returning it to distributors to use for different means rather than throwing it away. Every day, edible would-be food waste from stores is picked up and donated to soup kitchens. They even donate the scraps to animal rescue centers, literally repurposing *all* of what would otherwise be discarded.

- **Atlas Brew Works** is an innovative, Washington, DC–based brewery that has partnered with the Environmental Working Group (EWG) to make a rescue

> ### Did You Know?
>
> "One of the most common arguments people seem to have at home is about whether or not food should be thrown out just because the date on the label has passed. It's time to settle that argument, end the confusion and stop throwing away perfectly good food," Representative Chellie Pingree said.[20]
>
> The Food Date Labeling Act aims to standardize food date labeling and simplify regulatory compliance. It seeks to require all food manufacturers to use just two standardized labels: "best if used by" to indicate quality, and "expires on" for safety. It also calls for consumer education to help Americans better understand date labels; the allowance of the sale or donation of food past its quality date; and cooperation between the US Food and Drug Administration (FDA) and the US Department of Agriculture (USDA) in standardizing the labels. The key goals are to provide consumers with clarity so they can save money and cut back on wasting good, safe food.

beer called Ugly and Stoned out of unused stone fruits. All the proceeds go to EWG.

- **Tesco** is a grocery store chain that's breaking the mold—less than 1 percent of their food goes to waste, and they're aiming for a zero-waste policy by 2018. They have also started a "food waste hotline," which suppliers and growers can call to point out areas of the supply chain where unnecessary waste is being perpetuated, so they can work together to find a solution.

Initiatives such as these are so inspiring because they reflect the true beauty of this movement, which occurs when we uplift one another. As we nurture and sustain ourselves, creating a sense of health and balance, we have so much more to give, and can begin to renew and inspire our immediate communities and eventually the world at large.

A healthy lifestyle is about your environment, your community,
and the people you choose to surround yourself with.
—Dan Buettner

Coming Together

Sometimes it can be hard to let go of certain foods, even if these foods aren't healthy or sustainable, because we've channeled all the fun and enjoyment of food into dishes that come at the expense of our health. We have emotional attachments to certain foods because we associate them with family, childhood memories, and cultural traditions. But it's becoming increasingly easy to access food that's both celebratory *and* healthy. This can actually help us create new traditions that can be even more meaningful. Figuring out how to work within the cultural customs—sparking innovation within the context of your own world—is half the fun.

There are countless ways that we can band together to create new activities, new traditions, and new memories. We're seeing local community centers and public areas

ECOfy: How Can You Reduce Food Waste?

- Make a weekly meal plan and a corresponding grocery list so you can buy exactly what you need.

- Only cook what you know you're going to eat. This is where checking in with your body before preparing a meal comes back into play. Take a moment to pause and honestly evaluate how much food your body will need, and cook accordingly.

- Use everything. We often cut off and throw away perfectly edible, tasty, nutritious parts of produce. There's no reason to discard broccoli stems or sweet potato skins—in fact, stalks and peels tend to be incredibly nutrient-dense. And even though you might not want to eat carrot peels or onion trimmings, you can use them to flavor a soup.

- Bring leftovers home from restaurants. My husband makes fun of me, but I always enjoy them the next day!

- Turn leftovers, or produce that's slightly wilted, into a casserole, stir-fry, or soup.

- Buy seasonally when possible—it's a safe bet that seasonal produce won't have traveled as long before arriving in your kitchen, so it will stay fresh longer.

- Buy "ugly foods." Most supermarkets throw away the left-behind produce. So do your part by repurposing some of this. Buy some ugly tomatoes and use a blender to make a healthy bowl of gazpacho. Purchase apples to turn into applesauce. You don't need pristine produce, as it all looks the same in the blender.

- Participate in co-ops. There are plenty of opportunities to buy from local co-ops along with your neighbors. They often source from local farms and offer healthy and organic food to your community.

- Donate your extra food to a shelter. Ever find yourself throwing away boxes of food during your spring cleaning? Set that food aside and take it to a local shelter so they can feed those in need.

- Composting is the best way to repurpose food waste.

host farmers' markets, cooking classes, educational courses, and larger-scale events such as cooking competitions. Each of these events brings the community together through food, allowing locals to dig in while socializing and enjoying the festivities.

Celebrations of the ECOrenaissance food movement are happening all around us, every day.

Farm-to-table restaurants. The farm-to-table chef is a new form of restaurateur, one who understands how his or her vision impacts the local environment and surrounding world. More and more chefs want to know who's farming the food they're serving diners, and are unwilling to receive prepackaged produce and meats from an industrial manufacturing plant. "Farm to table" means that food is obtained directly from the person producing it without passing through an intermediate supplier. In addition, farm to table ensures that ingredients are seasonal.

This movement creates connections and collaborations through direct sales relationships, community supported agriculture (CSA), farmers' markets, and local distributors, empowering the collective, and making people emotionally closer on a level beyond social and business interactions. Think of the wonderful connection that occurs as the chefs have the opportunity to visit the farmers, walk around the farmland, and even pet the animals and sample the produce before they order it. Forming relationships with local farmers and nature itself infuses a much more meaningful connection into the purchasing of food, and sourcing seasonal ingredients dramatically widens the palate and expands creative culinary possibilities.

Food trucks. Food trucks are also driving the ECOrenaissance, as they facilitate a community atmosphere whereby potential customers wait in line and chat about their day while food is served from a truck. Because of the low cost of operation, many food truck owners get to focus their attention on chef-driven menus that offer diners a glimpse

Food Festivals

In the spirit of gathering to enjoy healthy and delicious ECOrenaissance food, there are now festivals entirely devoted to the celebration of good food. Some standouts include:

Eat Drink Vegan
Outstanding in the Field
Panorama
Seed Wine and Food Festival
VegFest

into the owner's heritage, family recipes, food vision, source of ingredients, and cultural cuisine. These trucks can be seasonal, adaptable, and flexible in their menu offerings. This flexibility gives owners the ability to connect directly with consumers, as the food is cooked and often served by the chef herself or himself.

Food trucks are also centerpieces of festivals, from small, local food and culture festivals that bring together all sizes of communities to large-scale music and arts festivals that attract people from around the world.

Food halls. The food hall movement enables your senses to travel all over the world. Food halls are springing up in many cities, where purveyors are able to both save money and create community by sharing kitchens and seating space. Since the vendors aren't financing the location, they're able to spend the extra money productively, by channeling it toward higher-quality food, including the use of more organic ingredients. This kind of innovative dining experience is disrupting the mentality of financial gain at the expense of health and sustainability.

The food hall movement has enabled exposure to and participation in food experiences that would otherwise be too costly or physically inaccessible for many people. An absolutely amazing and cutting-edge conscious food hall I just discovered is Copenhagen Street Food, launched by visionary restaurateur Dan Husted.

Creating Community Around Conscious Eating

- **Host a vegetarian cookout or a make-your-own vegan pizza party.** For a cookout, you can make (or buy) delicious plant-based patties—black bean and quinoa or sweet potato and wild rice are two simple and delicious examples, and Beyond Meat offers hard-to-tell-it's-not-meat plant-based alternatives. And be sure to try Good Catch tuna-free burgers and sliders or crab-free cakes! For plant-based pizza, you can buy or make a pizza crust, slather it with tomato sauce and your favorite spices and herbs, and then load up on veggies and vegan cheese from Follow Your Heart, Miyoko's, Heidi Ho, or Daiya.

- **Plan a plant-based potluck.** On a weekly or monthly basis, get together with your fellow foodies, and have everyone bring their favorite healthy dish. As you inspire and learn from one another, you'll start empowering each other to go further in your exploration of mindful, conscious eating. (Refer to the food blogs and cookbooks in the plant-based section of this chapter for ideas.)

- **Have a healthy scavenger hunt.** With your friends/kids/partner, make a list of your ten favorite snack foods and desserts. Seek out their plant-based, certified-organic alternative or try making your own.

- **Visit your local farmers' market with family and loved ones.** This can be a great way to bond and connect with others, especially in the summertime. Often there are live music and delicious samples. It's like going to a festival celebrating local, seasonal food. Farmers' markets are all about community and collectively supporting local, independent growers and farmers who really care about what they grow and sell to the public. To find a farmers' market near you, look at these websites:

  www.ams.usda.gov/local-food-directories/farmersmarkets
  www.localharvest.org/farmers-markets/
  www.farmersmarketonline.com/openair.htm

- **Order door-to-door delivery for your family and/or friends.** These are just a few of the many organic and plant-based (option) delivery services rocking the ECOrenaissance:

  Blue Apron—www.blueapron.com
  Forks Meal Planner—www.forksmealplanner.com
  Green Chef—www.greenchef.com
  Purple Carrot—www.purplecarrot.com
  Thrive Foods Direct—www.thrivefoodsdirect.com
  22 Days Nutrition—www.22daysnutrition.com
  Veestro—www.veestro.com

- **Join your local food co-op.** Typically, in exchange for a few hours of work per month, co-op members receive significant discounts on fresh, seasonal, local produce. Being part of this offers a chance to connect with a local community around food, learn about growing seasons, and gain access to affordable local food. (To look up your local co-op, go to coopdirectory.org.) NCG national co-op (www.ncg.coop) is a prime example of an ECOrenaissance grocer, offering all-natural foods across thirty-eight states.

- **Become a member of a CSA (community-supported agriculture).** This is a fantastic way to support local farmers. When you connect with a CSA, you purchase a regular share of several varieties of seasonal vegetables from a local farm; the vegetables will be delivered either right to your doorstep or to a convenient nearby pickup location. Generally, members pay up front for an entire season, which secures the farmers' ability to purchase equipment, new seeds, and everything they will need to grow the most holistically nourishing produce. To find your local CSA, go to www.justfood.org/csaloc and search by zip code.

- **Tune in to a food podcast:**
    Bite
    Food Heaven
    Gastropod
    Good Food
    MindBodyGreen
    Real Food Mamas
    Real Food Whole Health
    The Sporkful

When consumers begin to notice where their health is being compromised, they can begin to make better choices. The more awareness we bring to the issues at hand, the faster we will see change.
—Vani Hari

In the end, an ECOrenaissance lifestyle is both a rebirth and a lifelong process. Perhaps you're already well into your journey, and this information serves you as a reminder of the interconnectivity of food and the importance of eating consciously. Maybe all this is new to you, in which case, be patient with yourself. Recognize that shifting your relationship both to food systems at large and to your own sense of individual health, in a way that's sustainable *and* regenerative, will nourish and fulfill you throughout your life.

As a culture, we are beginning the much-needed process of looking at food as a kind of preventative medicine, as a means of restoring and renewing the health of the earth and our bodies. When it comes to food waste, toxicity, and scarcity, the world is in a crisis. The faster-cheaper-more mentality we have been operating under comes with consequences, and we're currently living with the repercussions. We've normalized imbalances such as disease, depression, and anxiety, but these are not our natural states. Broken food results in broken health: "dis-ease." To generate the abundance we deserve and to heal the world, we have to lean in and listen to the intuitive wisdom of all that nature has provided us.

> When it comes to food waste, toxicity, and scarcity, the world is in a crisis. The faster-cheaper-more mentality we have been operating under comes with consequences, and we're currently living with the repercussions.

The ECOrenaissance is all about no compromise, and when it comes to food, we now have access to a wealth of innovative and exciting options. Be curious and playful—experiment with recipes, do your own research, get in tune with what nourishes your body fully, and allow you to be your best self. Practice compassion—for yourself, for the earth, and for all creatures that inhabit our planet. Have fun with food, and watch in amazement at the transformation that will occur in and around you.

The DNA of ECOrenaissance Food: No Compromise in Taste, Health, or Ecology
- Certified Organic/GMO-free ingredients.
- Plant-based over animal proteins.
- Support local (farm-to-table) sourcing.
- Whole foods with minimal processing.
- Conscious eating; connection to food as energy.

- Minimize food waste at every opportunity.
- Regenerative, not degenerative, agricultural practices.
- Avoid fake-, fast-, and factory-farmed.
- Create delicious *and* nutritious meals.
- Use healthy food to create community.
- Share, support, and collaborate with loved ones around better food choices.

Illuminartist Interviews: *Food*

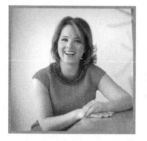

Ashley Koff, Licensed Dietitian

www.ashleykoffapproved.com

You may have seen this dynamic dietitian on the *Dr. Oz Show*, sharing her passion for better—not perfect—nutrition. Tune in to her podcast *Take Out with Ashley and Robyn*.

What is a personal ECOrenaissance tip you can share with readers?

Better nutrition *better be delicious*—choose foods more often that delight your senses as opposed to food products that check nutrient boxes.

What is your vision for the future of food?

The sum of the parts is always better, not perfect, so I envision a world where we each bring our best more often, and celebrate each other for it.

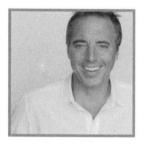

Dan Buettner, Author/Founder of Blue Zones

www.bluezones.com

Dan has literally found the formula for living longer with his brilliant global study on the world's blue zones. Explore his amazing work, as it will be well worth the trip.

What is a personal ECOrenaissance tip you can share with readers?

The blue zones share nine lifestyle tenets that create an environment of health; we call these the Power 9. "Right Tribe" is one of the easiest ways to make the world a better place because it's something we all do already: spend time with friends. The world's longest-lived people chose, or were born into, social circles that supported healthy behaviors.

Okinawans created *moais*, groups of five friends who committed to one another for life. Research shows loneliness is contagious, so by creating powerful friendships we can all live longer and stave off loneliness even in old age.

How did you start your journey toward sustainability/social purpose?

It all started in the spring of 2000 when I was leading a series of educational projects called quests in which a team of scientists investigated some of earth's great puzzles. I had heard about Okinawa's unusual longevity a few years earlier and thought it would be a great quest to investigate their secrets to good health and long life. We spent ten days studying, exploring, and summing up what we found. Five years later, I returned to Okinawa with a new team. I'd just written a cover story for *National Geographic* called "Secrets of Long Life," which profiled three areas of the world with concentrations of some of the world's longest-lived people—areas we dubbed "blue zones." I was determined to delve deeper into the lifestyle of Okinawans. During these explorations we were always thinking about how we could bring these teachings back to our communities. This is how the blue zones project was born. We decided that we could take the nine evidence-based common denominators that we found in all the blue zones and implement them in communities across the United States. Our goal was to make small adjustments to make the healthy choice the easy choice for people in their communities.

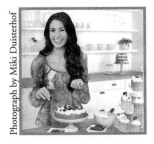

Photograph by Miki Duisterhof

Chloe Cascarelli, Chef/By Chloe
www.chefchloe.com

With five cookbooks and a creative, cutting-edge restaurant chain she founded, Chloe is at the forefront of cool and conscious plant-based eating. Follow her on Instagram!

What is a personal ECOrenaissance tip you can share with readers?

Shop smart. The world is at our fingertips—use the Internet to find out what ingredients and materials the products you consume are made of. If you can't find a compassionate choice for the products you want to purchase, demand one. Thanks to the Internet, we can let our consumer voices be heard without even leaving our homes!

Which of the pillars of the ECOrenaissance movement (collaboration, consciousness, community, creativity, connection) resonate most with you and why?

Collaboration is key for making change. As they say, teamwork makes the dream work. Even better, surrounding yourself with a team that's working toward the same goal, the same future, the same renaissance is what will move mountains. For me, collaborating with my mom daily over recipes and flavor combinations is a building block for my success.

What is your vision for the future of food?

The future of food is vegan; of that I am sure. Our food system will not sustain itself otherwise, so it's up to the chefs to step up their vegetable game. Luckily, consumers are getting hungrier and hungrier for innovative veggie burgers and almond milk lattes, so the future is looking bright!

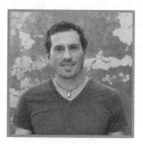

Gunnar Lovelace, Founder of Thrive Market/Love Heals
www.thrivemarket.com
www.loveheals.com

Gunnar embodies good leadership on every level. Intelligent, articulate, and inspiring, Gunnar is driving a true food revolution delivered right to your door. Become a member of Thrive Market!

What is a personal ECOrenaissance tip you can share with readers?

In an era of increasing political cynicism, those with a desire for authenticity and transparency continue to realize the growing power of voting with our dollars.

What is your vision for the future of food?

As the desire to access organic, non-GMO, and fair trade continues to explode, more innovation and holistic capitalistic values will be driven into the marketplace at scale. It's imperative for the future of our species and the health of our planet that we change the way we produce, distribute, market, and consume food.

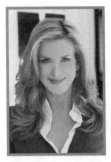

Kathy Freston, Author/Wellness Activist

www.kathyfreston.com

Kathy's beauty and passion have graced her cookbooks and restaurant collaborations, making plant-based eating stylish, sexy, and sustainable. Follow her work!

What is a personal ECOrenaissance tip you can share with readers?

Eat plant-based protein rather than animal-based foods! Animal agriculture is the leading cause of species extinction, causing 18 percent of all global warming gases (and that's conservative; World Bank scientists say the number is closer to 51 percent), uses one-third of the earth's land to grow crops that cycle through animals, and is the leading cause of water pollution. As for human health, too much animal protein raises the likelihood of cancer, heart disease, type 2 diabetes, and obesity. In addition, our callousness toward the animals we raise for food diminishes our humanity.

The great news is that there is so much clean protein available to us: beans and legumes, nuts and seeds, meat alternatives such as "chik'n" and veggie sausage, tofu and tempeh. There are tons of cool restaurants that are devoted to vegan food, as well as forward-thinking mainstream restaurants that have really hearty, delicious options alongside the traditional animal-based fare. This kind of shift makes us healthier and kinder as individuals, which ripples out and makes the world a better place to live in!

How did you start your journey toward social purpose?

I became obsessed with how to make the shift easy for people. I'd struggled with it myself, so I knew what the hurdles were, and I just kept addressing things in a way I would have appreciated when I was trying to figure things out. I figured that if I—being the meat-loving southern girl I was—could make the move away from eating animals, anyone could. I just had to communicate respectfully and warmly, as I would have wanted to be approached when I was learning.

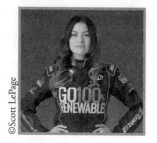

Leilani Munter, NASCAR Driver
www.leilani.green

A road and planet warrior like no other, Leilani will blow your mind and heart as she drives a better and more sustainable future for all. Watch the film *Racing for Extinction*.

What is a personal ECOrenaissance tip you can share with readers?
Make your next car electric, put solar panels on your roof if you can, and go vegan.

How did you start your journey toward sustainability/social purpose?
I hold a degree in biology from the University of California at San Diego specializing in ecology, behavior, and evolution, but I've been concerned about the human impact on the planet since I was a young girl.

Which of the principles of the ECOrenaissance movement (collaboration, consciousness, community, creativity, connection) resonate most with you and why?
Consciousness. The kind of life you choose to lead is defined by the moral choices you make every single day; make choices you can be proud of.

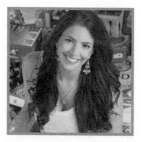

Vani Hari, Founder of foodbabe.com/*New York Times* Bestselling Author
www.foodbabe.com

Vani has taken the food world by storm with her authentic and tenacious cool-factor-meets-activism; check out how just one woman has made a real difference.

What is a personal ECOrenaissance tip you can share with readers?
Every time you purchase a product, you're sending a message to the manufacturer that says, "I support what you're doing." When we vote with our dollars, we not only help strengthen the companies that are doing the right thing by supplying healthy products

and sustainably grown food, but we also send a clear message of disapproval to those companies that are putting harmful products into the marketplace. By sending a clear message of what we want, we're actively shaping the marketplace around us.

How did you start your journey toward sustainability/social purpose?

I often refer to myself as an accidental activist because I didn't grow up thinking I was going to be one. I just wanted to feel better; I was tired of being sick all the time and wanted to take back control of my health. Once I began investigating what was in my food and uncovering the truth about the food I had been eating, I knew I had to share what I had learned. The information I uncovered about the food industry was so appalling that I had to speak out.

What is your vision for the future of food?

More and more Americans are waking up to what has been done to our food: a REVOLUTION is happening and will continue! More and more consumers are asking for healthier food without fake chemical additives, flavors, colors, preservatives, pesticides, and GMOs. Consequently, there is a landslide of artificial additives falling out of our food, and progress is happening across the industry. I envision a world in which the industry finally meets the consumer's demand for nontoxic, sustainable, and organic products while shameful practices (such as factory farming) cease to exist.

4

It's All Well and Good

When we heal the earth, we heal ourselves.
—DAVID ORR

Visualize for a moment: you go into your bedroom and close all the doors, windows, and vents. While you're in this enclosed space, you're smoking cigarettes, spraying Lysol and Clorox, chemical hair sprays and beauty products, and painting the walls with conventional paint. Can you still breathe?

Waste from food in your room starts rotting, and plastic packaging starts piling up because it has nowhere to go and doesn't break down. As the environment around you grows increasingly poisonous and unlivable, how do you feel?

This may seem like a hypothetical example presented to make an important point, because no one in his or her right mind would actively participate in this type of behavior. When we shrink our living space and limit our breathable air, it's easy to imagine the impact of a toxic environment on our physical and mental health. Our planet is much larger, but it's also contained.

Now, imagine flinging open the doors and the windows, with a renewed appreciation for the fresh, cooling air that floods your system. That air is coming from the very ecosystem that we are naturally blessed to have. We can't destroy that home. Trees and oceans create oxygen that we breathe in to survive.

What will happen when we can't open the windows? How will this impact the lives of loved ones such as our children? Or even our beloved household pets—our cats and dogs? We're just starting to see the tremendous environmental impacts of our consumer choices. If we don't make sensible and considerate changes now, our children, grandchildren, and great-grandchildren will suffer deeply from decisions they didn't make and actions they didn't take. In fact, I just returned from New Delhi, India, where the air quality was ten times worse than the government's acceptable pollution level, so the room I had you visualize felt all too real. I literally couldn't breathe.

> If we don't make sensible and considerate changes now, our children, grandchildren, and great-grandchildren will suffer deeply from decisions they didn't make and actions they didn't take.

The state of our home, our work space, and our social spaces have a very strong connection to our physical, mental, and spiritual state. And it goes without saying that *we* have a clear impact on our surroundings. We hold the power to curate a blissful, balanced space—or conversely, one that's chaotic and toxic.

Wellness is the convergence of mind, body, spirit, and space. In this chapter we'll go into depth on this concept, exploring our relationship with the earth and looking at how we can use nature's wisdom to heal our physical bodies and elevate our spirits, connecting back into all that is. Specifically, we start by focusing on the foundation for all life: water and oxygen. Together we will discuss how the water we drink and the air we breathe can impact our basic and fundamental health. We need clean air and water to exist, yet humanity remains the greatest threat to our ability to maintain them. It's important that we shift our actions both individually and collectively to become protectors of what is actually at the core of our very own survival.

As we build strong roots and a balanced environment for our body, we can then extend this practice to our mind and spirit, which are often lost in the shuffle of our sometimes obsessive emphasis on our weight and appearance. This chapter will also explore the connection between body and mind by showing exactly how they both coexist in space, which is an external factor that can absolutely impact our health. With that said, let's start with a single drop of water, then dive deeper.

> The way you eat, how you spend your money, the way you
> vote, as well as the way you relate to the environment itself,
> are determined by your compassion and willingness to see
> how your individual actions impact the collective whole.
>
> —Seane Corn

Water for Wellness

Water is a powerful reminder of how inextricably tied we are to nature. Not so coincidentally, it both makes up 70 percent of the human body and covers 70 percent of the earth. We feel so connected when we're in and around water. We experience a sense of beauty and freedom when we're at the beach, feeling the waves lap against our skin. We love the peaceful bliss of a still lake. We feel a deep calm listening to the sound of rain falling. And who doesn't love a hot, calming bath when we're stressed out? I'm truly in awe whenever I'm connected to this healing element. In art, literature, and many religious and spiritual practices, water is a powerful symbol of cleansing and rebirth.

Water is the essence of our vitality. We can't survive without it. Our brains are made up of 95 percent water, blood is composed of 82 percent, and the lungs contain 90 percent. Just a 2 percent drop in our body's supply can trigger signs of dehydration. But as our society continues to engage in harmful, careless practices that pollute the oceans and deplete our global water supply, access to clean water is dwindling at an alarming rate. Our own human wellness is dependent on the wellness of the oceans. But with plastic vortexes, mercury pollution, and destruction of underwater ecosystems and coral reefs from coal burning and the acidification of our oceans, our sources of life are growing more and more toxic.

> As our society continues to engage in harmful, careless practices that pollute the oceans and deplete our global water supply, access to clean water is dwindling at an alarming rate.

To sustain human life and protect the vitality of the earth itself, we need to seek solutions. Let's look at some of the ways

Try This: How to Hydrate Sustainably

- **Reducing water waste:** On average, each American uses ninety-eight gallons of water every single day—more than seven times what we actually need. Small daily actions actually do make a difference. Some examples:

  1. Turning off the tap while brushing your teeth or while washing dishes.
  2. Shortening your showers (and washing your hair less often—which actually is much better for your hair anyway).
  3. Minimizing the use of garbage disposals (which require lots of water to run properly).
  4. Using dishwashers and laundry machines only for full loads.
  5. To take it one step further, consider investing in water-efficient household appliances for showers, dishwashers, laundry machines, toilets, and faucets. Efficient technologies (such as WaterSense) can save 18 percent more water than conventional appliances, both conserving this crucial resource and cutting down on water bills.[1]

- **Reducing or eliminating plastic:** As much as possible, commit to living without bottled water and other plastic packaging. Plastic is extremely destructive to the oceans and all the ecosystems that dwell within, as it doesn't biodegrade—if you haven't already, look up pictures of the Pacific Garbage Patch and check out 5Gyres.org to learn more about the Texas-size pile of plastic pollution floating in the ocean. Plastic is also harmful to human health. It often contains BPA, which has been found to interfere with hormone function. Carrying a reusable and/or stainless-steel water bottle such as a S'well bottle (they're doing some really cool, stylish, and fun collaborations; see www.swellbottle.com) with you everywhere makes it simple to avoid disposable plastic bottles. It's the safest, most harmonious way to stay refreshed and hydrated. If you're caught in a situation where you do need to buy a plastic bottle, always look for BPA-free packaging.

- **Cutting down on or eliminating meat and dairy:** You may remember from the previous chapter that animal agriculture—*especially* livestock—is incredibly resource-intensive. One gallon of milk takes a thousand gallons of water to produce, and a pound of beef takes twenty-five thousand gallons of water to produce. Taking shorter showers to reduce water waste is a no-brainer, but eating one hamburger is the equivalent of showering for two months straight!

you can preserve water in your daily life—as well as some incredible innovations happening around water conservation, purification, and even creation.

Creating Water out of Thin Air

In truly solution-driven, innovative ECOrenaissance fashion, my friend David Hertz has developed a technology that literally creates fresh, clean water out of thin air. According to the US Geological Survey, there is more fresh water available in the atmosphere than in all the rivers in the world put together. David's company, Sky Source, uses "atmospheric water generators" to capture condensation from the air and turn it into water.

According to Sky Source's website, www.skysource.org, "Each Skywater 300 model is capable of producing up to 300 gallons of fresh water per day, enough for a household or emergency relief efforts, and can do so more efficiently than any other method of moisture extraction or filtration. Smaller models, such as the Skywater Harmony, are capable of producing drinking water on demand, perfect for home or office use.

"The machines use refrigeration techniques to maintain a dew point within a condensation chamber to maximize water production from the existing atmospheric condition—the higher the humidity and temperature, the more water that can be produced. After condensation, the water is filtered and treated with ozone to enhance its taste and prevent potentially hazardous microorganisms from forming."

While today David's machines may not be accessible at a mainstream level, I believe that innovations such as these are just the beginning of a new potential chapter in protecting water, one of the earth's—and humanity's—most valued and critical resources.

Just Breathe (Clean Air)

Breath, like water, is a powerful symbol of our relationship to nature. We share the air with every living creature on this planet. We even share air with plants—trees essentially "breathe" through the chlorophyll in their leaves. Through this process, they absorb much of the carbon dioxide in the atmosphere, cleaning and purifying the air. We breathe in the oxygen that trees create for us. We can't survive without the breath of plants.

But as we continue to harm our environment, perpetuating mass deforestation and polluting the very air we depend on for our basic existence, we no longer experience the full benefits of this natural exchange. A clean environment means clean, fresh air circulating through our bodies. To sustain our source and keep our bodies pollution-free, it's important to think about the ways in which we can reduce pollution and contribute to cleaner air:

- Choosing to bike or walk instead of driving.

- Cutting down on or eliminating meat and dairy—or going fully plant-based. Animal agriculture is responsible for more than *half* of greenhouse gas emissions.

- Purchasing clothing from thrift stores or eco-friendly companies rather than fast fashion chains, as *fast fashion is the second-largest polluter in the world, after coal.* (We will discuss this in much more detail in chapter 6, on fashion.)

- Keeping potted plants in your living space can help oxygenate a room. (Also, regular exposure to nature in any amount is shown to have extremely positive mental health benefits.)

- Using eco-friendly cleaning products from companies such as Seventh Generation, ECOS, Method, and Jessica Alba's The Honest Company. Conventional household products are typically quite toxic and are huge contributors to air pollution, so substituting eco-friendly cleaning products—or making your own—can have enormous health benefits for both your body and the environment. Which brings me to . . .

I'm a big believer in doing small things every day, because those tiny habit shifts will add up to big changes over time.
—Michele Promaulayko

Creating a Sanctuary: ECOfy Your Home

A healthy home is where it all starts. We *are* our environment. Our most intimate space, our home, can make or break our sense of health. Let's look at how we can draw inspiration from our larger home to create a clean, green sanctuary in our living spaces.

Bring the Outside In

In our society, it's easy to forget that human beings are not separate from nature. We thrive in natural environments. Studies have shown that natural scenery has enormous mental health benefits. But we don't really need studies to tell us this—think about how you feel when you lie on a field of grass, or dive into a lake, or take a hike in early spring when flowers are blossoming. When we immerse ourselves in nature, we feel alive and at peace. Create a similar sensory environment in your home by buying fresh flowers and tending to potted plants or a small garden. And being able to see nature from your window can dramatically enhance your well-being.

My friend Danielle Posa is the creator of the online brand the Wellbeing Hacker.[3] Her work consists of developing online courses, public speaking, and leading corporate workshops—all focused on the topics of well-being and conscious leadership. Her work reminds us of our connection to the world around us. She says, "We've grown up in a society that leads us to believe that humans are separate from nature instead of showcasing the ways in which we're very intricately connected.

"Because my focus is on elevating people's well-being and quality of life, I highlight the research that supports how this connection with the natural environment is impacting our brain, body, and overall feeling of being alive. In my opinion, when we make it clear to people how much the natural world is serving us in these ways, we're less likely to ruin it."

Check This Out

An excellent and informative article from *Slate*, "Gazing at Virtual Nature Is Good for Your Psychological Well-Being."[2]

I asked Danielle to outline some ways to reconnect with nature. Here are some of her favorite tips and tricks:

- **Wander, wonder, daydream, and daze.** Soft fascination is what occurs when we're mesmerized by the movement of waves, a flickering fire, a swaying of trees, or a running waterfall, and it has been proven to create a calming effect on the mind. This happens because of the combination of the ever-changing yet consistent nature of these moments, which can stimulate the mind. This one concept, in my opinion, provides us with a great excuse to take those much-needed pauses in life, enabling us to be present in the beauty all around us. So allow yourself to be caught up in the moment, releasing yourself from any other intention. Wander through the forest on your hike—not because you're trying to get a workout in, or to see how fast you can finish your hike—but simply for the sole purpose of wandering. Stare at the waves or the clouds, gently observing their movements and shapes.

- **Fill your home with plants, natural light, and pictures of water.** Studies show that each of these things boosts your mental state. Even just a picture of an aquatic scene can affect your mood. Plants have been proven to reduce stress and anxiety.

- **Don't just go outside, find the cleanest air.** With the majority of the population living in cities, it's hard to find clean air there. Truly "clean air" is full of negative ions that neutralize free radicals, enhance our moods and immune systems, and balance our autonomic nervous systems. They also clear the air of allergens and bacteria. Indoor air, even in an air-conditioned room, lacks these negative ions and can often lead to headaches, nausea, and stress. So get out there, ideally among the trees, or near naturally flowing water. This is the air that's most soothing to your mind and body.

- **Take breaks from computer screens and phones.** Our addiction to our screens is known to increase depression rates, and the more we're glued to our screens and phones, the less we're making time for the outdoors.

- **Take your shoes off and get dirty.** We live in a hypersterilized world. We've been trained to fear germs, and to clean our hands at every opportunity. And yet this is proving to have the reverse effect on our health. We're killing our natural bacteria and therefore weakening our body's natural ability to heal itself. We've got to allow ourselves to get dirtier. Take your shoes off. Walk around outside barefoot so you can feel the earth and stimulate parts of your feet that are usually so overly protected. Or start that garden. Plant some seeds with your bare hands. Physically connecting with the earth as opposed to constantly protecting yourself from it is a great way to break the facade of separation.

Aromatherapy: Sensuality Meets Wellness

Nature invigorates our senses in a number of ways. Investing in an aromatherapy diffuser can be a great way to bring the fragrances of plants into our home. Breathing in the rich scents of essential oils (make sure they're organic) can have a number of effects, from deeply relaxing (lavender, chamomile, sandalwood) to energizing and vitalizing (lemon, grapefruit, orange, basil, rosemary). But the powers of essential oils go even further—they can be harnessed as remedies for many common ailments.

Healing properties of essential oils
- **Lavender oil** for healing burns and cuts and soothing insomnia.
- **Peppermint oil** (mixed with a base oil such as argan or coconut) to soothe sore or tense muscles.
- **Clove oil** has antibacterial properties and is especially useful for fighting oral conditions such as cold sores or canker sores.
- **Eucalyptus oil** improves treatment of respiratory conditions and allergies. (You can also hang a bunch of fresh eucalyptus in your shower to help clear congestion when sick.)
- **Rosemary oil** improves brain function and memory. It also can thicken hair, so it's a great addition to shampoos.
- **Rose oil** reduces inflammation and makes the skin glow.
- **Ginger oil** reduces inflammation and relieves nausea.

Essential oils are also more eco-friendly than candles, which are often made from palm oil and synthetic materials.

My favorite organic essential oil companies are:

Auracacia
AVEDA
EO
I AM fragrance
Intelligent Nutrients
Jurlique
NOW foods
Thrive Market

Clean and Green

The microenvironments we create in our homes are mirrors of the earth. Nothing is separate.

Did You Know?

Essential oils have so many benefits, from natural fragrances to healing properties. But did you know that certain essential oils can actually act as aphrodisiacs? Damiana is one such oil. Check out the new brand Flor de Amor, which celebrates this intoxicating hero ingredient. Damiana comes from a small shrub native to Mexico and Central and South America and has a soft citrusy, floral smell. It has been found to increase oxygenation and blood flow to sexual organs in both men and women. Plus, once the lights are dimmed and the lush aroma of Damiana is stirring your sensual side, reach for a Sustain condom, which uses eco-friendly, nontoxic materials and fair-trade labor. Who says sustainability isn't sexy?

- **Seek alternatives to conventional toxic paints and carpeting.** Did you ever wonder why when you paint your home, or get new carpets put in, it smells so bad you can barely breathe? A lot of people don't really think about it, but you can go to Home Depot and find an eco option. Or visit ecobuildingproducts .com, which is like a mini green Home Depot, to look for sustainable, breathable options.

- **Avoid toxic cleaning products.** Read the backs of conventional cleaning products and google them—it's shocking that these products don't come with warning labels. Many people are turning to more natural products once they have kids and witness the detrimental health effects firsthand. But there's no right time to start going green; it's never too late or too early.

- **Cut down on disposables.** Replace Ziploc bags with glass containers, Tupperware, or Mason jars; substitute old dish towels for paper towels; and use cloth napkins and nice utensils instead of flimsy plastic versions. Switching to these sustainable choices will create a subtle elegance in your home while saving money as one-time buys. Win, win, win!

- **Green your sleep.** On average, we spend about one-third of our lives sleeping. But now, cutting-edge home textile and loungewear companies are making it possible to be an ecowarrior twenty-four hours a day. Buying organic sheets offers an easy (and important) first step to greening your home. Dr. Mercola (www.Mercola.com) offers certified organic sheet sets and is also coming out with the ultimate green sheets, which protect your body, and the planet, while you sleep. They're called "shielding sheets," and they're made of a silver filament that naturally repels electromagnetic energy. They're also made with organic cotton and nontoxic finishing (I will expand on the importance of this in chapter 6). With organic cotton bedsheets now available from Farm to Home (farmtohomeorganic.com) to QVC to luxury brands such as Coyuchi and Boll & Branch, there's no reason to buy anything *but* organic cotton bedding if you truly want to sleep peacefully and dream of a better world. Did you know that there are nearly two pounds of toxic chemical pesticides in the cotton it takes to make just one nonorganic bedsheet?

Creating wellness in your home is not just limited to the household products you use. It extends to the furniture you purchase, the manner in which they're manufactured, the materials they use, and even how they're delivered to your home. As you introduce these structures into your living space, you're simultaneously interacting with potentially harmful products. Susan Inglis is executive director of the Sustainable Furnishings Council (SFC) and is a resident expert with the organization she helped found in 2006.[4] She has led SFC to work with industry leaders to establish criteria to gauge the sustainability of furniture products and practices; develop programs for educating all sectors of the industry; and attract hundreds of companies to membership.

We spoke about the value and importance of sustainable and healthy furnishings in your home. Here's what she had to say:

Furniture is complex! Pieces are often made of many different materials, many of which might be processed using harmful chemical inputs, some of which may still be present when the furniture comes home. Asking what it's made of will help you avoid a few chemicals that may be particularly harmful, including flame-retardant chemicals, fluorinated stain treatments, antimicrobials, PVC, and VOCs, including formaldehyde. When it comes to a material such as wood, the most important consideration is that the wood should be legally harvested from well-managed forests, ensuring the health of the forests we depend upon to absorb our CO_2 emissions, as well as to supply wood for future use. Look for legitimate third-party certification, such as by the Forest Stewardship Council (FSC), and for reclaimed material.

I then asked her how consumers can make smart purchasing decisions. She shared her wisdom:

- **Be a conscious consumer.** Transportation is a major contributor to greenhouse gases. Look for furniture that was made closest to where you live, using materials that are also from your region. Buying local will not only cut emissions but also support your local economy. Manufacturers that take good care of their people empower communities to take care of their environments, too. Look for a company's code of conduct to be assured that workers are fairly treated, paid decent wages, and work in a safe environment.

- **Avoid products with harmful chemicals.** Textile production accounts for more toxic waste pollution of water than any other industry. Harmful chemicals are used in growing the natural fiber or creating the synthetic fiber, in processing it into thread, in making the fabric, and in finishing the cloth. You can reduce the amount of toxic chemical inputs by choosing organically grown fibers and by looking for certifications of safe manufacturing.

- **Find energy-efficient appliances.** The production of electricity is the single largest contributor to CO_2 emissions worldwide. Always seek energy efficiency in the products you choose. But even if the product does not draw energy in use, consider what it took to make it. Solid and simple materials are more energy-efficient than complex ones. Further, companies with an energy-use reduction plan are a significant part of the solution.

- **Shop SFC members**. Companies that have made their own verifiable commitment to sustainability. For free guidance to hundreds of sources, visit www.sustainablefurnishings.org.

Don't forget, home is where the heart is, so have fun creating your own inspiring "home, sweet home."

Avoid using chemicals in the home! You may not have control over your surroundings at all times, but everyone has control over their home!
—**Shannon Beador**

Home Is Where the Healing Is: Natural Remedies

Growing up, my kids almost never got sick. They were in touch with their bodies, and intuitively connected to nature and its healing potential. Now I watch my twenty-year-old son and twenty-two-year-old daughter looking online for natural, herbal remedies when they're feeling off-balance—and it puts a huge smile on my face. Sometimes, no matter how we take care of ourselves, imbalances (and accidents) strike. We just have to know how to nurture them from a holistic place.

- **For nausea:** Ginger in any form, including tea, works wonders on an upset stomach.

- **For allergies:** Eating a spoonful of raw, local honey every morning can assuage seasonal allergies.

- **For colds and flus:** Apple cider vinegar can be made into a tea (with honey and lemon), or, if you're brave, taken as a shot. It's an incredibly effective immunity booster—some people swear by a daily dose as a way to avoid colds and flus altogether. For something a little more mild, mint tea with lemon and honey soothes many of the symptoms.

- **For cuts and open wounds:** If you get a cut, take the cellulosic lining on the inside of an organic eggshell and apply it to the cut—all the nutrients will absorb into the skin, and it seals the open wound as an adhesive. This can be an amazing way to avoid both Band-Aids and stitches. In my family, we call this the "egg trick."

- **For digestive issues:** Take digestive enzymes (my favorite brand is Enzymedica) and probiotics (my faves are Renew Life and Garden of Life). So many people have digestive issues such as bloating and constipation, and these enzymes and probiotics are incredible for helping your body optimize digestion, absorb nutrients, and convert food into energy. If you have to take antibiotics, make sure to take digestive enzymes and probiotics to help rebalance your system.

- **For sleep issues:** I take a magnesium supplement every night before bed—magnesium plays a huge role in calming the nervous system. I also try to sleep in complete darkness and quiet, and if necessary, I wear earplugs and an eye mask. There are so many soothing, relaxing remedies for sleep issues—a calming bath with lavender spray (or rubbing lavender oil on your temples) or a cup of chamomile tea can work miracles. Additionally, don't go to bed angry or upset, which affects your emotional well-being; and try to get movement or stretching in during the day so that your body is prepared for rest. We have lots of work to do to heal our planet and our lives, so make sure you get the sleep you need!

Going with the Flow

For some women, menstruation is a source of real discomfort. And until a certain age, of course, periods can't be avoided. But by improving diet and exercising regularly, we can alleviate a lot of the uncomfortable symptoms that can accompany our cycles. Sugar can really exacerbate cramps, headaches, and mood swings. And switching our feminine products can make quite a significant difference, too. Studies have shown that using organic, nonsynthetic menstrual products can alleviate many of the common symptoms associated with that time of the month.

Note that as of yet, the FDA does not require conventional tampon/pad companies to list their ingredients, so we don't really know what we're putting in direct contact with our most delicate, sensitive areas. Purchase a DivaCup, or pure, unbleached, organic cotton pads/tampons from companies such as LOLA (started by two millennial women with a mission to infuse transparency into feminine products), Cora, Seventh Generation, Sustain, Natracare, or Jessica Alba's The Honest Company. DivaCups or organic cotton products are not only a much safer choice for our bodies, they're also infinitely more eco-friendly than their conventional counterparts.

Holistic Health Is Intuitive

No matter how much it gets abused, the body can restore balance. The first rule is to stop interfering with nature.
—DEEPAK CHOPRA

Contrary to what the current condition of human health might lead us to believe, wellness is our natural state. Our bodies have innate balancing mechanisms, just like the larger forces and ecosystems in nature. When we are truly in tune with ourselves, we're typically more in tune with the world around us. Our bodies are just microcosms of our earth's macrocosm. In the spirit of the ECOrenaissance, the more conscious, creative, collaborative, and connected we are from within, the clearer it becomes that from our individual selves to our local, regional, and global communities, we're all one. When we grasp that concept, we can understand how our own thoughts, behaviors, and actions can influence human and planetary wellness, and ultimately the greater good.

> When we are truly in tune with ourselves, we're typically more in tune with the world around us. Our bodies are just microcosms of our earth's macrocosm.

Think about the force of nature in our own intuition. For example, what makes pregnant mothers naturally hungry for foods rich in the specific vitamins that they need? And it's this innate ability that also allows us to, say, walk into a troubled conversation and immediately sense the tension in the air, it's "so thick you can cut it with a knife." There's a reason why we describe that tension as being palpable enough to cut. We can physically feel it.

Many of us are conditioned to tune out the amazing powers of perception that we're born with, instead of having this innate resource nurtured and developed. This causes us to grow up disconnected from our bodies and from nature. The first step toward lasting personal and planetary wellness is connecting back to the intuitive knowledge that we all possess.

Try This: Trusting Your Inner Wisdom

- Do you ever hear a voice inside that seems to be giving you a different answer from what someone may be telling you? Pay attention to that voice.

- Have you ever thought about yourself in relation to nature . . . that humanity has evolved as part of, not against, our environment? Walk barefoot. Breathe in the air with your eyes closed.

- Do you ever feel inexplicably drawn to a person you've met that you want to know better? Find a way to connect with him or her.

- After eating, do you feel a difference depending on the types of foods/meals you've selected? Start journaling and note these differences.

- Have you felt uncomfortable, or perhaps your skin broke out, after applying a new personal care product? Read the label, and if it's a bunch of long words you don't understand, start exploring new products with healthier ingredients that will make you feel radiant.

- Have you ever watched a film, looked at a piece of art, or listened to a song and felt moved but stopped there? Go deeper and learn about its inspiration, and why it struck a chord for you.

> Wellness is about taking care of the whole, not the isolated parts.

In an ECOrenaissance mind-set, where wellness is about balance and awareness, taking care of ourselves means something different every day. Think of your entire being as an ecosystem. Infinitely complex, dynamic, and unique, your ecosystem is made up of your physical body and its state of health, as well as all the other internal and external factors that make you *you*—your mind, your emotions, your relationships, your soul, and your environment. Wellness is about taking care of the whole, not the isolated parts.

When we abandon one part of our personal ecosystem, we can feel it. We know in our gut that something is missing. Think about when you feel most balanced, energized, awake, and at peace. You don't feel that way at random—most likely, you feel that sense of serenity because many internal and external factors are converging.

Let's look at some of the holistic ways we can tune our ecosystems to the frequency of vibrant health, by looking at the whole picture.

Living Long, Living Well

My friend Dan Buettner, in his acclaimed book *The Blue Zones*—a book about pockets of the world where people live the longest and have the highest vitality (with the highest populations of "centenarians")—defined common lifestyle denominators in these areas:[5]

- Simple, local, plant-based diets
- Regular physical movement incorporated into daily life
- Spending time in nature
- Uplifting social interactions and a feeling of community
- A sense of spiritual or religious meaning
- A sense of purpose

The most important takeaway is that holistic wellness and longevity don't just refer to the physical, but instead they embody the convergence of every aspect of our lifestyle choices. If you're interested in learning more, Dan has a fantastic TED Talk that delves further into his findings.

- **Eastern medicine:** Have you ever tried acupuncture or Reiki? Both are super-effective treatments to help clear your body and align your mental/emotional and physical states. Acupuncture addresses imbalances in the physical body by examining and treating the root of the problem rather than the isolated symptoms. And Reiki goes deep by treating the energetic body. Personally, I do my best to seek out holistic treatments for any physical imbalances, and I avoid pills whenever possible. "Modern medicine" has its time and place, of course, but ultimately it's a Band-Aid, treating physical symptoms and not the root cause. (Of course, as with everything, there are exceptions.) Feel like disposing of some of the medications you no longer are willing to use or those that have expired? Be careful not to just flush them down the toilet or toss them in your neighborhood sewer. Many expired or unused medications enter our water sources through irresponsible disposal practices. A study conducted by the US Geological Survey found measurable amounts of one or more medications in 80 percent of the water samples drawn from a network of 139 streams in 30 states.[6] As I've mentioned before, when we listen to our bodies and embrace holistic wellness that's in tune with our inner and outer environments, physical ailments are suddenly few and far between.

- **Earthing:** As I've learned from Dr. Joseph Mercola (sign up for his amazing newsletter at Mercola.com), simply put, "earthing" means physically connecting to the earth. It's based on the idea that many of our health conditions (anxiety, depression, insomnia, fatigue, high blood pressure, diabetes, asthma, cancer, and Alzheimer's, to name a few) are rooted in our modern disconnect with the earth, its subtle rhythms, and its innately healing energy. Earthing can be as straightforward as taking regular walks barefoot. The key is grounding into the earth with no human-made barriers (such as shoes). Earthinginstitute.net offers this explanation for the importance of skin-to-earth contact: "The body is mostly water and minerals. It's a good conductor of electricity (electrons). The free electrons on the surface of the earth are easily transferred to the human body as long as there is direct contact. Unfortunately, synthetically soled shoes act as insulators so that even when we're outside we don't connect with the earth's electric field. When we're in homes and office buildings, we're also insulated and unable to receive the earth's balancing energies."[7] You can find more ways earthing can help you fight disease at draxe.com/earthing/.

- **Mindfulness:** Mindfulness originated as a Buddhist practice, focused on staying centered in the present moment. Recently it's been embraced by larger demographics in the West as people look for deeper connections in life. There's a lot of buzz around the concept of mindfulness, but at its core it simply means slowing down and paying attention. Mindfulness can be applied to breathing, eating, walking, listening, observing—really, anything we do can be done mindfully. But in spite of its simplicity, this practice can be a game changer. It grounds us in our bodies and in the world, and heightens our awareness and powers of perception. Mindfulness empowers us to discover that we have all the answers inside us if we just listen. It reminds us of who we really are, on the individual *and* global levels. How do you feel when you drop in to nature? When your toes are in the sand or the ocean at the beach? When you're hiking in a forest? When you're smelling a flower? Do you think about how your consumption habits are affecting others and the world around you? Take stock of your choices, appreciate what you have,

Did You Know?

A recent *Huffington Post* article explains the science of mindfulness. Focusing on the work of Ohio State University psychologist Dr. Ruchika Prakash, this article describes how mindfulness can serve as a useful framework for understanding how to improve brain health. Dr. Prakash says, "The way we're thinking about mindfulness both in terms of cognitive health and brain health ties into the adaptability of different networks in the brain." Dr. Prakash found that four weeks of mindfulness training could reduce "emotional dysregulation" among multiple sclerosis sufferers, for example—an important finding, considering that 50 percent of chronic disease patients experience some form of depression.[8]

and recognize that your day-to-day actions (and inactions) can truly make a difference.

Care about where your "stuff" comes from. Who made it? Who suffered for it? How were they treated? When those answers are more important than our need to look a certain way, the world will change for the better.

—**Maranda Pleasant**

Self-Care

Self-care is any action that feeds us on a spiritual level, refueling and revitalizing us in a profound way. I have several go-tos when I need to refuel. I love to get massages—they're not only so effective physically but they also harness the emotionally/spiritually healing power of touch as a reminder of our interconnection with others. A professional massage is wonderful, but even a massage from a partner or a friend can do the trick. And despite my busy schedule, I always try to make time to get outside and walk around. I'm a huge vitamin D advocate— sunshine makes me feel invigorated, and walking rejuvenates me.

Here are a few other suggestions for self-care practices:

Connect: Taking Action

The ideas of waste, water pollution, and climate change can affect our state of mind. Joining in as a steward of the environment can actually empower and nurture us on a very deep level. Check out some of these incredible environmental groups that may excite and empower you to take action:

Climate Reality Project
Environmental Defense Fund
Environmental Working Group
Global Green
Greenpeace
Natural Resources Defense Council (NRDC)
Nature Conservancy
Safer Chemicals, Healthy Families
Sierra Club
350.org
World Wildlife Fund

- Find a volunteer position or hobby doing something you love.

- Join a common interest group such as a creative writing, photography, or pottery class. Creativity feeds our souls and helps us connect to the world around us.

- Slow down your mornings and nights—don't go to sleep angry or stressed, and don't rush into your day. Take time each night before bed to truly unwind, and time in the morning to start your day off with positivity, gratitude, and intentionality.

- Meditate. Pausing to connect to breath is one of the most essential self-care actions, as it reminds us of both our fundamental humanity and our relationship with all that is. Breath moves through all living things, and we're part of this dynamic and synergistic exchange.

We need to move away from seeing our own well-being, liberation, and happiness as selfish pursuits—quite the opposite! Our society can only move forward if it is composed of conscious, thriving individuals. At its best, wellness is a conduit for helping us live our fullest, most enhanced, and most meaningful lives. And as we experience the abundance that becomes inevitable when we're fully tuned in, we indirectly give others permission to step into their own light, their own truth.

Love doesn't know how to stay within the lines, so it's going to have some interesting pivots, twists, and turns, but love is creative and unstoppable, and it makes the impossible possible.

—Robyn O'Brien

Curated Community Wellness Spaces

The power of community to create health is far
greater than any physician, clinic, or hospital.
—MARK HYMAN

Community spaces are a vital piece of the wellness equation. No matter how much you revel in your personal journey, you'll probably find yourself looking for others to share it with—conscious peers and friends to celebrate the process with, mentors and teachers who will gently guide you forward and remind you of what matters, healers of all sorts who will help restore your body, mind, and spirit to balance with nature. And now these community spaces are cropping up in abundance. In fact, in early 2018, my company became a founding member of a new conscious work space model in New York City called the Assemblage (www.theassemblage.com). This cutting-edge community work space offers complementary organic and vegan meals for members, stimulating evening events, and yoga and meditation classes daily. Now that's motivation to go to the "office"!

Meditation Studios

By now we've all heard of and even discussed the incredible benefits of meditation for both mental and physical health (to name a few, it lowers stress; boosts immunity; improves sleep; enhances mind/body connection; heightens awareness; and improves memory, clarity, and focus). However, I've spoken to many people who feel a little intimidated by meditation—for some, the word conjures up austere images of sitting in total stillness in a perfect lotus pose in front of an altar. But at its core, meditation is just bringing consciousness back to breath, which connects with the life source that runs through all things. You can meditate anywhere and in any pose—my favorite time to meditate is actually on airplanes. I find it incredibly soothing to be soaring through the clouds, physically removed from the everyday noise of my life. Check in with yourself to see what resonates for you. A bath or sauna session? A hike or bike ride?

For the modern meditator, drop-in studios seem to strike the perfect balance between the internal process of meditation and the advantages of being part of a community. These studios bring meditation communities together, providing a common space for anybody wishing to practice mindfulness.

One innovative example is Inscape, a multiplatform meditation brand that has invented a novel way to access meditation: Inscape is both a studio in New York City and an iOS app, empowering consumers by giving them the choice of where, how, and when to practice meditation. Inscape is just one example, but drop-in meditation studios are a fast-growing trend in cities. Below are a few others:

- New Mindful Life (San Diego)
- Meditate (Chicago)
- The Den (Los Angeles)
- Unplug (Los Angeles)
- MNDFL (Manhattan)

To find a meditation studio near you, go to meditationfinder.com. If you can't make it in person, check out these apps and websites:

- Headspace
- Smiling Mind
- Buddhify
- Jiyo
- The Mindfulness App

Meditating Our Way to a Better World

The value of the practice of meditation is being recognized far and wide. Prisons, hospitals, veteran support initiatives, and offices alike are offering daily meditation sessions for the various healing benefits to be gained. Schools replacing detention with meditation are also seeing transformative and inspiring results.

W. Coleman Elementary in Baltimore is one such school, where instead of punishing disruptive kids or sending them to the principal's office, they're invited to visit the Mindful Moment Room instead, which is filled with lamps, decorations, and plush purple pillows. Kids are encouraged to sit in the room and go through breathing practices, helping them to calm down and recenter. They're also asked to talk through what happened and think about their actions, as well as find alternative solutions for the next time.[9]

Think about how the world would be different if we all meditated daily, and if all the institutions and organizations we were part of began to implement the practice of meditation. We would all likely become calmer and more connected beings. We would be grounded in the right ways, while likely not allowing our emotions to quickly grow into anger or resentment. We would have better ideas, since we would then be using a greater level of brainpower in our daily activities. We wouldn't be as distracted, and could focus more on meaningful connections with those we love. We would be happier, as meditation reduces depression, anxiety, fear, and nervousness. In short, we could perform at happier, higher, and healthier levels . . . if we just meditated. The ECOrenaissance calls for this greater sense of connection, empowering all of us to greater levels of existence.

High-Vibe Group Movement

Movement is our birthright. It's an essential piece of the wellness puzzle. When we move our bodies in an intentional, joyful way, the physical meets the spiritual, and we tap into something profound and essential. It transcends the practice itself, reflecting our desire to go deeper. Exercise is no longer just about one-dimensional satisfaction—people are seeking movement modalities that will touch their lives on multiple levels. Following are my top three ECOrenaissance choices, all of which facilitate community and fuel consciousness:

- **Ecstatic Dance Movement:** A substance-free, curated DJ experience where people gather to experience the pure, electric energy that accumulates when we drop in, let go of constraints, dance intuitively, and move around and with one another. The Get Down in New York City is an absolutely contagious ecstatic dance experience if you get to the area. Or for your own journey, you may want to download the soulful grooves of one of my favorite DJs, DJ Sol (www.djsol.com), whose music is positively invigorating on every level.

- **Soul Cycle:** An intense, spiritual-meets-physical, full-body experience. From the website: "At Soul Cycle we believe that fitness can be joyful. We climb, we jog, we sprint, we dance, we set our intention, and we break through boundaries. The best part: We do it together, as a community" (www.soul-cycle.com).

- **Yoga:** My personal favorite way to move my body; the core intent of yoga is to connect breath to movement. Yoga for me is a time to reflect internally, breathe most deeply, and rejuvenate my body and soul in an unparalleled way. I find that the mat is one of the only places where I can truly turn off the volume on the virtually constant mental noise.

The practice of yoga isn't new, of course. But it's exciting to watch how much it has expanded—from an obscure, hippie-dippy concept in America to an all-out craze (which, to me, shows just how far we've come in a short span of time). Yoga can mean many different things to many different people, and there's now something for every*body*, every need, and every mood.

- High impact: Power Vinyasa or a hip-hop yoga class (Y7)
- Focus and rigor: Hatha, Iyengar, or Ashtanga
- Deep, slow stretch, breath, and energy flow: Yin or Kundalini
- Unwind: Restorative or Sivananda
- Or, if you can't make it to a studio, take advantage of the wealth of free, full-length yoga classes online.

Through the practice of yoga, I became more mindful, and cultivated the necessary tools to heal from the limited beliefs that made me feel separate from people and the world around me.
—**Seane Corn**

Wellness Centers, Spas, and Resorts

Wellness is at the root of human beings feeling conscious, nurtured, and healthy. It's when our spirit is broken, our bodies are blocked, and our minds are cloudy that we can't see the light we carry within.

In this global movement for wellness, spas are shifting their focus from indulgence to connection. They're like charging centers for humans. I look at the spa experience as preventative medicine—going to and getting a massage in a spa is my version of a trip to the doctor. It's not just about feeling good, it's also about healing the body and awakening the mind and the spirit. (The Global Wellness Institute—previously named the Global Spa Institute—is dedicated to educating the public about preventative health and wellness.)

Many spas, recognizing the relationship between human and planetary wellness, are now "greening" their spaces for a fully immersive, connected experience (go to green spanetwork.org for a directory of these enlightened wellness centers). Some of my personal favorites include:

- Rancho Le Puerta in Baja California, Mexico
- Canyon Ranch in Tucson, AZ, or Lenox, MA
- Mohonk Mountain House in New Paltz, NY
- Miraval Resort & Spa in Tucson, AZ
- Mii amo in Sedona, AZ
- Travaasa in Austin, TX
- Ojai Valley Inn & Spa in Ojai, CA

Besides California, Arizona, and Texas, you can find clusters of amazing yoga, spa, and eco-resorts in places such as:

- Tulum, Mexico
- Goa, India
- Koh Samui, Thailand
- Bali, Indonesia
- Costa Rica
- Palomino, Colombia (my new fave is Reserva One Love)

There has also been a rise in interdisciplinary wellness centers that fuse group classes such as yoga, movement, meditation, and wellness workshops with personalized services such as acupuncture, energy work, nutrition coaching, and massage therapy.

A few highlights include:

- Floating Lotus (Manhattan)
- Esalen (Big Sur)
- Exhale Spa (Manhattan, multiple locations)
- Maha Rose (Brooklyn)
- Lifetime (Manhattan, multiple locations)
- Wanderlust Wellness Center (Los Angeles)
- The Springs (Los Angeles)
- The Standard Spa (Miami)
- VigorMe (Miami)

So far these are being offered primarily in larger cities, but my hope is that they will spread quickly (very probable, as the wellness industry has been one of the fastest-growing industries of the past few years).

Online Wellness Communities

Want to be guided into a wellness journey? Seeking inspiration or holistic healing but don't know where to start or can't find an in-person space? Check out these inspirational podcasts, blogs, online courses, and thought leaders:

Podcasts
Bliss and Grit
Dharma Ocean
Liberated Body
On Being
Soul on Fire
That's So Retrograde
The One You Feed

Websites, Blogs, and Magazines

Goop
MindBodyGreen
ALIVE magazine
OneGreenPlanet.org
Organic Spa Magazine
ORIGIN magazine
The Numinous
The Wellbeing Hacker
THRIVE magazine
Well & Good

Online Courses

Chopra Center: Meditation, personal growth, mind-body, Ayurveda
DailyOM: Yoga, body love, creativity, rituals
Off the Mat and into the World: Yoga and activism
Shaktibarre (Sisterbiz coaching): Fitness and yoga, Ayurveda, chakra balancing, holistic counseling

Revolutionary ECOrenaissance Medical Doctors to Follow

Dr. Caldwell Esselstyn
Dr. Colin Campbell
Dr. Dean Ornish
Dr. Harvey Karp
Dr. Joel Fuhrman
Dr. John McDougall
Dr. Joseph Mercola
Dr. Mark Hyman
Dr. Michael Klaper
Dr. Neal Barnard

And finally, Dr. Scott Stoll, who is a bestselling author, Olympian, and international speaker with a vision and passion to inspire a new generational vision for health. He's the cofounder of the Plantrician Project and the International Plant-Based Nutrition Healthcare Conference. We spoke about wellness, and he offered this helpful prescription for all of us:

- We must shift our mind-set from ownership to stewardship. A steward values and views the world as a gift to be shared and an inheritance for our children to believe in: us and our over me and mine, investment over instant gratification, save for the future over spend for today, cultivating and creating over cashing in, simplicity and small footprint over extravagance, personal sacrifice over personal accumulation, and improving and regenerating over using and depleting.

- The greatest opportunity every day to induce change is in the moment we exchange our money for something.

- Your life will change when you decide to begin growing something you will eat. Keep it simple and plant a few herbs, or kale, in a window pot or small box. You will connect to the very beautiful and real nature of life and be inspired to learn more.

- Take the first two minutes in the morning when you open your eyes to begin your day with gratitude, reflecting on each part of your body, working from your brain to your toes.

- Support organic agriculture by purchasing organic food from local and national farmers, and give to organizations such as the Rodale Institute.

- Transform health care by first transforming yourself and your family through a healthy whole-food, plant-based diet and lifestyle, and then when your health-care practitioner asks about your healthy changes, share your story, as personal testimony is a powerful tool. Use documentaries such as *Forks over Knives*, *Eating You Alive*, *What the Health*, and *Game Changers* as easy entry points, and support organizations that are educating healthcare practitioners, such as the Plantrician Project and the Physicians Committee for Responsible Medicine.

- Engage the children in your life to value environmental stewardship by studying the origins of the food we eat, clothes we wear, cars we drive, relationships we share, and our place in this world and history. Make it fun: visit places such as farms, factories, and animal shelters, grow a garden, and volunteer to help those in need.

- Eat plants with gratitude, learn about the benefits of the food you eat, make food delicious, and share a meal with family and friends every day.

ECOfy: Take Action

Contribute to your own wellness by asking questions such as:

- Do my daily responsibilities leave me feeling stressed, anxious, or nervous?
- Do I wish I spent more time each day quietly in thought?
- Do I put down my cell phone, turn off the television, and truly disconnect enough?
- Am I finding myself more irritable or tired lately, causing me to be cynical instead of optimistic?
- Am I spending enough time with my family and friends, ensuring I have a strong work/life balance?
- Do I do the things I love, taking time for myself and enjoying my hobbies and interests?

These are all important questions to consider. If you find yourself negatively answering any of these questions, it makes sense to dive a little deeper and consider why. These are all directly related to your personal wellness, and you might not be focusing enough time and energy on your mind/body health. You simply cannot compromise your physical, emotional, and spiritual well-being. If you do, you will eventually burn out and find yourself trying to catch up and recover, which can actually be a vicious cycle.

We're at a pivotal time for humanity and the earth. Our survival requires deep love and care that can transcend our greatest challenges, stresses, and negative habits. As we awaken together in this ECOrenaissance, embrace the realization that we're connected to one another and our environment. Envision a path to collective consciousness that's clean and green on a holistic level so we can create an experience of wellness beyond our wildest dreams.

Remember, personal wellness is not a luxury, it's a necessity. Dr. Stoll outlines a great path for us all. It doesn't take a lot of money or even a substantial amount of effort to introduce wellness into your life. You don't have to invest in outside classes or instructors to meditate, practice yoga, or connect with your inner self through some quiet time. It's as simple as finding a peaceful space in your home, backyard, basement, garage, or even a local park. Make it your own if you can. Hang pictures, introduce music, and light incense. Set the mood for focus, and share it with your family and friends. Add this time to your schedule, and thoughtfully make sure you're spending a few minutes on yourself each and every day.

We're stronger in numbers and can build faster. I want to experience this collaboration on a worldwide scale.
—**Yogi Cameron**

The *Ultimate* Space: Our Planet

If our clutter and mess are piling up, we can streamline our home for a peaceful sanctuary. If we're feeling down, we can take a group fitness class or dance the night away, getting that rush of endorphins and forming new conscious friendships. If stress is becoming overwhelming, we can rejuvenate body, mind, and soul with a holistic retreat or a trip to a spa.

But at the end of the day, we can't take a vacation from Planet Earth. It's our one true home. Think about your relationship to the spaces around you, how you treat them, and how they treat you in return. Think about how nature moves you. How weather impacts your mood. How you feel when you move your body naturally and intuitively. How you connect to other living beings, whether those are soft and furry or green and leafy. What makes you feel grounded, balanced, and whole?

Well-being is our human right. Just like it's the right of flowers to bloom and trees to grow and animals to run around freely. Yet we're depriving ourselves of our birthright because we're so caught up in the material, constructed world. Let's look to the balance of nature, return to our intuitive knowledge, spread the energy of love—and thrive.

Global wellness starts at the individual level. Your well-being matters. The love, awareness, and balance you cultivate within yourself can make a real difference.

Global wellness starts at the individual level. Your well-being matters.

Like begets like; we perpetuate abundance through the energy of celebration and appreciation. Knowing this, you may not be surprised by all the people you draw toward you as you progress on your wellness journey. You're not "just" improving your own relationship with the earth and fulfilling your greatest desire for happiness, you're also inspiring and activating those around you. Wellness is contagious, and can spread faster than almost anything else—a ripple effect that helps the ECOrenaissance movement flourish exponentially.

The DNA of ECOrenaissance Wellness: No Compromise in Physical, Emotional, or Spiritual Health

- Be conscious of the interconnections among mind, body, and spirit. Start and end your day with deep breathing to bring awareness to the balance between your internal and external self, and the world beyond you.
- Eat as healthily as possible; consume more plants.
- Exercise and move your body every day—with others, whenever possible (sex, walking, yoga, dancing, etc.).
- Sleep at least six to eight hours per night. Resting your body will bring the clarity needed to dream of a better world.
- Meditate at least five to thirty minutes per day. Imagine a greener, cleaner, and more mindful world.
- Find a place in your home and make it your own. Relax and reflect on how you can be a champion for positive change.
- Live mindfully with simple pauses throughout your day—slowing down and being present in the moment. Appreciate every breath you take, and thank our environment for sharing in this experience.

- Practice daily: affirmations, gratitude, balance, self-care, prioritizing, trusting your gut, and letting go of fear. You *can* achieve what you believe.
- Embrace love and community at every level (work, family, friends, etc.).
- Be one with nature.

Illuminartist Interviews: *Wellness*

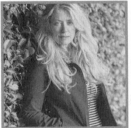

Maranda Pleasant, Founder of *Origin*, *Thrive*, and *Mantra Wellness* Magazines
www.originmagazine.com/www.mythrivemag.com/
www.mantramag.com

This power woman has used her art to create the ultimate ECOrenaissance community. Maranda's inspiring magazines have literally changed the face of publishing and can now be found online and on the shelves of countless stores nationwide. Truly good reading.

What is a personal ECOrenaissance tip you can share with readers?

The number one choice we can make for a cleaner, sustainable, more compassionate world is eliminating meat and dairy from our diets. With everything we know about factory farming, and its impact on climate, water, and animals, we can't be environmentalists and still consume animal products. Care about where your "stuff" comes from. Who made it? Who suffered for it? How were they treated? When those answers are more important than our need to look a certain way, the world will change for the better.

Which of the pillars of the ECOrenaissance movement (collaboration, consciousness, community, creativity, connection) resonate most with you and why?

Creativity is powerful. It drives radical self-awareness, thoughtfulness, and independence that for me leads to connection and community. Self-realized women creating is the most powerful thing on the planet. We birth movements for social change, art that moves people, urging others to rise. This much-needed revolution is born from freethinkers and creators who refuse to conform. Birthing change, pushing boundaries and edges, and protecting women are where the change makers live. I want to be there beside them.

What is your vision for the future of food, media, and/or lifestyle?

My vision is that media will rise up for love and protection of women and girls against bullshit narratives built to oppress us, attack our body, confidence, and beauty. We must stop comparing women, starving them, and keeping the focus on their outward appearance and not their inner strength and true beauty, which is the source of our power. Beauty and purpose only amplify as we age, and we need media to reflect that. We must communicate that a woman's worth is not dependent on how popular or liked she is, allowing her to rise up, become louder, unwavering, demanding change, until we all get it. A media role is in the revolution fighting for equality and change, and women are on the front line of that movement. Media has been used to suppress and marginalize women, and we are going to change that.

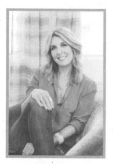

Michele Promaulayko, Editor in Chief of *Cosmopolitan*
www.hearst.com

A rock-star editor has the power to transform. This awesome woman, formerly the editor in chief of *Women's Health* magazine, has true vision and heart.

What is a personal ECOrenaissance tip you can share with readers?

I'm a big believer in doing small things every day because those tiny habit shifts will add up to big changes over time. It's easy to get daunted by trying to be perfect, and when that happens, we give up. So today it could be as simple as making sure the people in your life know which companies to buy from for your birthday or holidays. Tomorrow, you may decide to treat yourself to organic sheets and use your old ones as drop cloths. Don't hold yourself to 100 percent compliance on day one—that's too hard to live up to.

What is your vision for the future of fashion and lifestyle?

Each generation is becoming more informed about what goes into the products we use every day. Millennials and now Gen Zers feel strongly about patronizing companies that share their values—and they aren't afraid to boycott companies that don't. The accountability bar keeps getting raised, so the fashion and lifestyle industries will have to continue to evolve their practices to keep pace with these demands and win over the next generation of consumers.

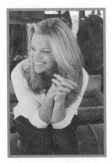

Robyn O'Brien, AllergyKids

www.robynobrien.com

A loving mother and a real advocate of Mother Earth, Robyn has inspired countless others to think differently about the choices they're making. Listen to her fabulous TED Talk.

What is a personal ECOrenaissance tip you can share with readers?

Share more—your heart, your clothes, your love. We have more than enough to go around. Share! If you've got a gorgeous ecowarrior outfit, share it, let others know how it looks and feels on them so that they can then turn around and become an ecoconsumer, too.

How did you start your journey toward sustainability/social purpose?

I got a late start. My awakening came after our fourth child was born. With her food allergy diagnosis, I became acutely aware of how important manufacturing and producing are—of food, of body care products, of cleaning agents, and of clothing and sheets. And I was on my knees in gratitude for those who had come before me, building out the products and companies to help keep her safe. Now, almost twelve years into it, I'm still profoundly grateful for all who have dedicated their lives to making the world a better place. We need all hands on deck!

What is your vision for the future of wellness?

My vision for the future is that this love story we're living—of healing our loved ones, our own health, one another, and our planet—plays out. It's being driven by an incredible awakening. It's happening at every level of our society: food, fuel, fashion, technology. It's an expansive, embracing, beautiful movement, and it is so love-fueled. Love doesn't know how to stay within the lines, so it's going to have some interesting pivots, twists, and turns, but love is creative and unstoppable, and it makes the impossible possible. Our lives are the love story, and it's beautiful watching it play out.

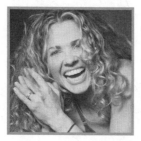

Seane Corn, Yoga Teacher
www.seanecorn.com

Seane is the living embodiment of yoga on and off the mat. Her beauty radiates from the inside out. Buy her yoga videos and join her vision for human and planetary wellness.

What is a personal ECOrenaissance tip you can share with readers?

If every person made a commitment to their own deep inner work, confronting the limited beliefs that often disconnect us from ourselves, each other, and the planet—whether it be through yoga, therapy, life coaching, getting into a twelve-step recovery program, or one of the many other ways to explore personal development and growth—the world would inevitably become a better place. The way you eat, how you spend your money, the way you vote, as well as the way you relate to the environment itself, are determined by your compassion and willingness to see how your individual actions impact the collective whole.

How did you start your journey toward sustainability/social purpose?

Through the practice of yoga, I became more mindful, and cultivated the necessary tools to heal from the limited beliefs that made me feel separate from people and the world around me. Yoga taught me to see the world around me as connected to the world within me, and that there was no separation between me, the perceived "other" animals, as well as the planet Herself. This understanding of interdependency impacted so many of my choices because I did not want to initiate any unconsciousness and felt a responsibility to not perpetuate behaviors that could hurt or harm the planet and those who inhabit it. Therefore my yoga practice led to becoming a vegan, my veganism helped me to understand the connection between factory farms and environmental injustice, my understanding of environmental sustainability led me to become more involved politically—so I could hold responsible the people charged with making policy and decisions that impact the planet directly.

What is your vision for the future of humanity?

My vision is that all souls wake up, do the inner work necessary, remember who we are and who we are to each other, love bigger than we ever imagined possible and live a life in service to love and God in all we say, do, and create. If we could do that, peace would be the inevitable outcome and we would coexist in a world that's free, safe, fair, equal, and loving for all.

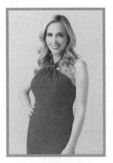

Shannon Beador, Reality TV Star, *Real Housewives of Orange County*
www.shannonbeador.com

Shannon is the real deal when it comes to her passion for living green. Leveraging her platform to inspire positive change, she stands out from the others in the *Real Housewives* series.

What is a personal ECOrenaissance tip you can share with readers?

If I could give one personal tip that would collectively make our world a better place, it would be to AVOID USING CHEMICALS IN THE HOME! You may not have control over your surroundings at all times, but EVERYONE HAS CONTROL OVER THEIR HOME!

Many people believe that when they purchase a product, the safest ingredients are used, but that's far from the truth. Most conventional household cleaning products are filled with chemicals. There are so many labeling loopholes that manufacturers don't include all chemicals used. Their toxic ingredients pollute the interior home environment.

Pesticides are regularly sprayed both inside and outside the home. Children play on the floors and on the grass, and most young children continually put their hands in their mouths. Our bodies are constantly inhaling the toxicity of the numerous pesticides used today.

But there is GOOD NEWS! There are natural alternatives. Homemade cleaning products can be mixed for pennies, and they do the job. There are so many natural remedies available to combat different pest invasions. And with the Internet, the answers can be found at your fingertips! How amazing is that? The natural alternative to household chemicals can eliminate toxicity and save you money at the same time!

How did you start your journey toward sustainability/social purpose?

My journey to healthy living began with the birth of my first child. I thought that all baby products were of course healthy for my child. My pediatrician, Dr. William Sears, started to educate me on the time frame for breastfeeding and when to introduce certain foods to avoid food allergies. I started to think. When I was young, no one ever spoke of allergies and asthma. Today it's commonplace.

I started to do some research and discovered that many things that were healthy in my childhood era are no longer healthy. (Now I'm dating myself.) Foods are processed, genetically modified, and filled with hormones and antibiotics, all in an effort to maximize profits.

I also discovered that the food industry was not the only arena using toxic ingredients to increase profitability. Most clothing, bedding, furniture, and building materials are not healthy. It's devastating that most consumers aren't even aware of the toxicity that they're exposed to on a daily basis.

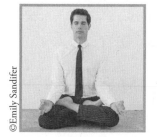
©Emily Sandifer

Yogi Cameron, Yoga/Meditation/Ayurveda Guru
www.yogicameron.com

If you haven't already bought Yogi Cameron's book *The Yogi Code: Seven Universal Laws of Infinite Success*, do so, as this former male supermodel may enlighten you on every level.

What is a personal ECOrenaissance tip you can share with readers?

Over the years we have become a "throwaway" culture. One positive habit we can cultivate is to buy the best quality of goods so we don't need to buy so much and end up throwing away so much. This is a more sustainable, eco-friendly model, which leads to a smaller carbon footprint as a way of living or lifestyle.

How did you start your journey toward sustainability/social purpose?

I went to study Ayurveda and follow the yogi path in India, and my guru would teach how first your mind and body need to be in balance before you can make balanced choices that are good for others and the ecosystem. This has made my life simple, sustainable, and much more purposeful. From here I can be of service to others while remaining socially conscious of the impact I'm having on the earth.

What is your vision for the future of humanity?

Building communities that have the same values and goals, that collaborate and grow as a unit and not as separate, competing entities. We're stronger in numbers and can build faster. I want to experience this collaboration on a worldwide scale. This is the new collective consciousness we're experiencing.

Surround yourself with people who bring out the best in you.
—RICHARD BRANSON

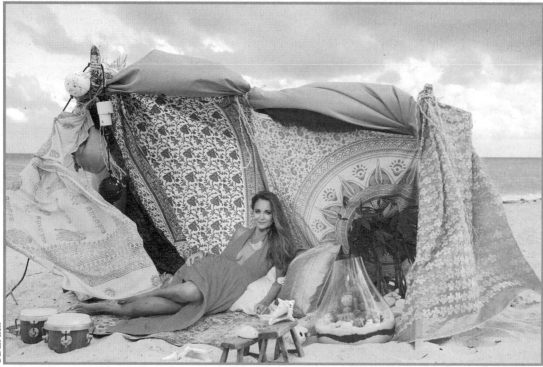

Feeling so good dressed in this naturally beautiful and cozy organic cotton sundress by one of my favorite conscious designers, Mara Hoffman. A bohemian fashionista basking at home by the sea at 1 Hotel South Beach, I'm radiating in Joanne Stone handmade hammered-gold earrings and her brilliant quartz bib necklace—truly responsible fashion with infinite meaning and beauty.

5

Beauty Inside and Out

If you have good thoughts, they will shine out of your
face like sunbeams and you will always look lovely.
—ROALD DAHL

Beauty is not just skin deep. True beauty starts at a deeper, soul level and radiates outward, engaging more than just the eyes. Sight is just one sense, and although our perception of beauty may start there, true beauty is a holistic experience, occurring when all the senses are in harmony. When we find something beautiful, it's because we're drawn to it in a way that transcends the aesthetic.

To make this more tangible, close your eyes and visualize the most stunning natural landscape you can imagine. Whether it's a snowy mountain, a misty meadow, a sparkling coastline, or a lush jungle—what does that image bring up for you? How do the colors and textures and smells illuminate your senses? What feelings does this image conjure? Serenity, comfort, awe, inspiration, excitement? We inherently recognize and connect with nature's beauty.

The ECOrenaissance movement is redefining what it means to be beautiful. It's a shift in philosophy, not your commonly accepted description. We're understanding that beauty is intrinsic and deeply felt, and we're moving away from the idea of beauty as nothing more than a surface trait, a widely accepted but flawed definition. Beauty is about authenticity, about connecting with the internal love and light that we all possess, and then sharing it outwardly with the world. It's about connection between internal emotion/thoughts and external purpose. The shift of the ECOrenaissance means connecting to the luminous beauty that we all possess. We are an extension of Mother Earth herself, and we're beginning to understand that true beauty comes from reconnecting with our essence.

> We are an extension of Mother Earth herself, and we're beginning to understand that true beauty comes from reconnecting with our essence.

Think of someone who absolutely radiates. We all know those people, who just have a glow to them—chances are, that person has tapped into a deeper, more meaningful, and more *alive* existence. We know it when we see it, and we know it doesn't come from a doctor or a tube. Think about your love for that person, and the happiness and transcendent beauty they bring to your life. You likely don't base these feelings on how they look or what they own. You might even feel this way because you have likely grown to know the heart and soul of that person, and value what's beneath the surface.

This is what beauty means in an ECOrenaissance context. We intrinsically understand people as beautiful when they're radiating positivity and love, and when they're comfortable with who they are at their core.

In this chapter we'll look at the ways the old standards have been harmful to human health (*especially* women's health) and environmental wellness, then explore how the industry is shifting for the better, and how we can all take beauty into our own hands through diet and lifestyle, conscious purchasing, and DIY products.

Beauty Leads the Way

It's undeniable that we're all drawn in by aesthetics. But we can use this to our advantage, to bring us toward a no-compromise understanding of beauty. What delights our senses can draw us into something deeper and be a catalyst for transformation.

Horst Rechelbacher, in his brilliant design for AVEDA, was a prime embodiment of this concept. He looked at beauty from the ground up, sourcing plant-based materials in a radical shift away from the traditional mind-set of the beauty industry. His products remind people where we come from, implementing pure essential oils and plant-derived ingredients, which function as herbal medicine. Horst avoided adding harmful ingredients to AVEDA products, instead incorporating only natural resources and loving energy.

Horst's father was an herbalist, and Horst grew up on an organic farm, engulfed in knowledge about the power of nature. AVEDA has always embraced the connection between food and beauty. Now it's fairly commonplace to hear people say, "If you wouldn't eat it, don't put it on your skin." But when AVEDA was starting out, that idea was unheard of.

Horst's iconic wisdom transcended his profession as a hairdresser and a creator of beauty products. He understood beauty in its truest form, as an extrasensory, full-body experience. He believed that behind all forms of beauty there is infinite unity, and this shaped how he sought to provide beauty through service, through love, and through an exchange of source energy that nourishes the soul. He taught me that true beauty is not an isolated characteristic, but a synergy between people and planet, between inside and out, and that our capacity to experience beauty gives us an unlimited potential to *create it* in our own lives and in ourselves.

People used to be convinced that beauty products needed certain chemicals to work, to stay on, and to maintain their color. But Horst put beautiful aesthetics first, so his stellar products continue to wake people up to a no-compromise beauty model. AVEDA broke major ground when it conceptualized plant-based beauty, but now so many brands have joined the plant-based, organic party.

Here are some of my favorite plant-based companies:

Personal Care
Acure
AVEDA
Beautycounter
Desert Essence
Dr. Bronner's
Dr. Hauschka
EO
Intelligent Nutrients
Jurlique
LotusWei
Tata Harper

Makeup
- AVEDA
- Bite Lipstick
- Gabriel
- Giovanni Cosmetics
- Honest Beauty
- Hynt Beauty
- ILIA
- Jane Iredale
- Josie Maran
- Mineral Fusion
- RMS
- Sante
- Tarte Cosmetics
- Vapor

When we inhale the rich scent of essential oils or nurture our natural beauty with pure products derived from minerals, we can feel the difference. Skin-care and hair-care products, makeup, and perfumes were invented to make people feel fresh, clean, glowing, and vibrant. Just imagine that you try on the most beautiful lipstick color you've ever seen, or sample a shampoo that smells like a field of lavender. You're already captivated—but then, imagine learning that the same product is also organic, locally produced, and made with love and integrity. It doesn't get any better than that.

When we pay attention to raw materials, whether it's ingredients, packaging, or textiles, and demonstrate honesty and accountability surrounding those choices— it makes a difference, and that's the future.
—**Kiran Stordalen**

What's Hiding in Our Beauty Products?

You've most likely either noticed the cultural shift toward a more natural look and simpler, cleaner products, or started implementing them in your own life. But the beauty industry has always gone through fads and trends. Is this just another temporary craze? What's *actually* so toxic about conventional cosmetic and personal care products? Let's pull back the curtain and look at the science of how conventional makeup as well as skin-care and hair-care products have been harming us and our ecosystem, and why we need to continue to turn toward green beauty.

- Our skin is our largest organ for absorption, so anything we put on our skin is being soaked into the bloodstream. Products such as birth control, nicotine patches, and other pharmaceuticals can be administered through the skin precisely because it's so permeable. In fact, many experts even agree that *absorption through the skin is more dangerous than ingestion by mouth.*

- Substances absorbed into the digestive system have the slight benefit of passing through our detoxification organs (the kidneys, liver, and colon), where enzymes help to break them down. Substances absorbed through the skin don't go through this process—they pass, unfiltered, straight into the bloodstream.

- Women are disproportionately exposed to these dangers. On average, American women use twelve beauty products per day, which translates into exposure to more than 168 synthetic, unregulated chemicals. And teenagers, who are using an average of seventeen products per day, are even more vulnerable to these risks.

- It's now being discovered that toxins in these products can even *pose a major danger to unborn babies.* The Canadian NGO Environmental Defense tested the umbilical cord blood of newborn babies and found that babies are now being born "prepolluted." They found that each child had been born with 55 to 121 toxic compounds and possible cancer-causing chemicals in their bodies.[1]

Sadly, many conventional beauty and personal care companies have overlooked these dangers, and most mainstream products are unnecessarily filled with chemicals and toxins. While developing AVEDA, Horst was in constant disbelief that conventional beauty products don't come with a warning label. Even today, in the United States, no policies have been enacted to eliminate—or even warn consumers about—the toxicity of our beauty products (while the European Union has completely banned hundreds of them).

Thankfully, resources do exist to help inform and educate consumers. Of all the potentially harmful ingredients we may find on labels, research has been done to prioritize the removal of key ingredients known as the "Mean 15." Adria Vasil, author of *Ecoholic Body*, takes us through the following ingredients, which pose the greatest risk to both human and environmental health:[2]

1. **BHA (butylated hydroxyanisole) and BHT (butylated hydroxytoluene):** The International Agency for Research on Cancer has listed these chemicals as potential carcinogens. They're not restricted in the United States, but California includes BHA on its list of chemicals that must be listed on product ingredient labels as potentially cancer-causing.[3]

2. **Coal tar dyes or PPD:** Coal tar dyes are very popular in the cosmetics industry because they provide rich, long-lasting hair color. But, like a lot of petroleum-based products, researchers claim that any degree of exposure can lead to health risks. Long-term use of these dyes can even lead to non-Hodgkin's lymphoma.

3. **Cyclomethicone and siloxanes:** If you like a clean windshield, dry underarms, or a smooth makeup base, you've probably used products containing siloxane. They interfere with hormone function and damage the liver. Environment Canada says that D4 (cyclotetrasiloxane) and D5 (cyclopentasiloxane) may build up in fish or other aquatic organisms. The European study reached a similar conclusion, rating the chemicals as "high concern."

4. **The ethanolamines (ammonia compounds) DEA (diethanolamine), MEA (monoethanolamine), and TEA (triethanolamine):** These unfriendly acronyms are found in creamy and foaming products such as moisturizer, soap, sunscreen, and shampoo. As cleaning product additives, emulsifiers, or foaming agents, these can be found in soaps and cleansers looking for an added

bubbly kick. They react to form cancer-causing nitrosamines, which are not only harmful to humans, but also to fish and other wildlife.

5. **Dibutyl phthalate:** It keeps nail polish from chipping, helps PVC remain flexible, and is used as a solvent for dyes and fragrances. But is it worth it? This chemical has been found to interfere with hormone function, especially during pregnancy.

6. **Formaldehyde-releasing preservatives (DMDM hydantoin, diazolidinyl urea, imidazolidinyl urea, methenamine, or quarternium-15):** These are widely used in hair and nail products and in moisturizers. They're used as preservatives in cosmetics *and* as active ingredients in some toilet bowl cleaners. Formaldehyde is *proven to cause cancer.*

7. **Parabens:** Widely used in makeup and moisturizers, parabens are a common preservative with links to impairing regular hormonal function. Studies have shown that parabens can mimic the effects of estrogen, which in an imbalanced state could lead to breast cancer for women and interfere with male reproductive function.

8. **Parfum:** Present everywhere, even in products marketed as "unscented" (it may also be listed as "scent" or "fragrance"). Parfum is actually not one single ingredient—it's a compound of many chemicals and, sometimes, essential oils. Since there are no regulations requiring companies to disclose the ingredient lists of their signature scents, the blanket term "parfum" is used. For people with chemical sensitivities, these unlisted ingredients can trigger allergic reactions, migraines, and/or cause asthma.

9. **Polyethylene glycols or PEG:** Widely used in conditioners, moisturizers, and deodorants, PEG can be contaminated with 1,4-dioxane, which may cause cancer. If perfectly pure, they're considered generally safe, though they're not recommended for use on broken skin. In rare cases, polyethylene glycol compounds can become contaminated with ethylene oxide—and that's when it gets really concerning. Ethylene oxide is a known carcinogen and can also cause developmental problems.

10. **Petrolatum or petroleum jelly (Vaseline):** It can keep skin hydrated, which is why it's often added to skin-care and hair-care products. But these products can easily become contaminated with carcinogens.

11. **Sodium laureth sulfate (SLES) and sodium lauryl sulfate (SLS):** They're common foaming agents used in dish soaps and foamy beauty products such as cleansers, shampoos, and bubble bath. SLES can be contaminated with 1,4-dioxane, which can cause cancer and liver damage. It can also possibly become contaminated with the known carcinogen ethylene oxide. *And* it can be harmful to fish and other wildlife.

12. **Triclosan:** Triclosan is a very effective antibacterial chemical found in lots of common consumer products, including toothpaste, hand sanitizers, laundry detergent, and facial tissues. Research has shown that triclosan sticks around in the environment long after we've finished using it, killing helpful algae and even accumulating in the bodies of other organisms.

13. **Retinyl palmitate and vitamin A:** A popular ingredient in acne serums, anti-redness, and antiaging creams, this ingredient smooths the skin at first, but under the sun it has been found to speed up the harmful effects of UV rays.

14. **Palm oil:** An edible oil used in processed foods and cosmetics, palm oil is linked to major issues such as deforestation, habitat degradation, climate change, animal cruelty, and indigenous rights abuses in the countries where it's produced, as the land and forests must be cleared for the development of the oil palm plantations. According to the World Wildlife Fund, an area equivalent to the size of three hundred football fields of rain forest is cleared each hour to make way for palm oil production. This large-scale deforestation is pushing many species to extinction, and findings show that if nothing changes, species such as the orangutan could become extinct in the wild within the next five to ten years, and Sumatran tigers, in fewer than three years.

15. **Oxybenzone (BP-3/benzophenone) and octinoxate (octyl methoxycinnamate):** These are two sunscreen chemicals that may disrupt our hormonal systems and that can trigger allergic reactions. Sunscreens containing zinc oxide, titanium oxide, and avobenzone are much safer.

At first, this amount of information may seem a little overwhelming, but there are many helpful tools to guide you on your journey toward incorporating sustainable, natural products into your life:

- **Environmental Working Group's Skin Deep database:** This is one of my favorite resources. They have compiled more than 64,536 products, so you can look up and learn about anything and everything in your bathroom or makeup bag. Just enter the product in question, or even a single ingredient of concern, and the site will generate a full analysis along with a toxicity ranking between 1 and 10.

- **Lily Tse's Think Dirty app:** The app was born of Lily's personal quest to understand the facts about products and labeling in light of her family history of cancer. In her research, Lily found that our overexposure to toxins from cosmetics and personal care products is linked to many forms of cancer. With Think Dirty, you can scan the bar code of a product or search for it by name. The app then provides you with a 1-to-10 toxicity ranking and up-to-date ingredient information as well as safer alternatives within each product category—and a direct link to Shop Clean.

The power is in our hands, as consumers, to demand more of this positive change—the more we move toward beauty products that are formulated from nature, with loving energy and with the greater good in mind, the more the industry will move away from conventional, harmful chemical formulas. True to the ECOrenaissance, we're driving a movement that only continues to grow. We're deeply connected to emerging beauty trends, and we have the power to redefine beauty for a better world.

The industry *is* shifting—that much is clear from the explosion of holistic beauty brands that have emerged in recent years and that are lining the shelves of your neighborhood pharmacies such as CVS, Walgreens, and Duane Reade. In addition to supporting more conscious brands, there are so many ways we can all take our health and beauty into our own hands, which we'll explore in the following pages.

The future of beauty is marked by cleaner products,
safer formulas, and significant innovation around natural
ingredients—with the customer calling the shots.
—**Gregg Renfrew**

The Skin-Gut Connection

In the ECOrenaissance spirit of interconnectivity, we know that looking good on the outside really does begin with your insides. Our external issues always have an internal root, and our skin is basically a mirror for our gut health. Figuring out what you can add to your diet and beauty routine—as well as figuring out what you may need to remove—is an exciting journey that begins with listening to the messages your body is sending you, experimenting a little, and using the health of your skin as a road map.

Favorite tips for radiant skin:

- **Support gut health** by taking a daily probiotic supplement. My favorite brands are Renew Life, Jarrows, and Garden of Life. Or drink your probiotics in a delicious Kevita Kombucha.

- **Eat more vitamin A–rich foods** such as sweet potatoes, carrots, oranges, and peppers to help skin cells overturn more quickly, avoiding breakouts.

- **Eat more high-quality fats** such as in avocados, flaxseeds or hempseeds, and coconut products.

- **Eliminate inflammatory foods** such as dairy, which can be a major cause of acne.

- **Lay off the synthetic skin products**, as their chemical makeup, aside from being a major health gamble, can really dry out your skin; even so-called moisturizers have this effect. And in some cases, this dryness can cause skin cells to overcompensate by producing excess amounts of sebum, leading to a greasy or oily face. Try a more mild, natural product, or moisturize with a light, balanced oil such as argan (my favorite brands are Intelligent Nutrients and Acure).

The Ultimate Beauty Food: Sea Greens

The key to feeling like a mermaid is eating like one! Seaweed—an incredibly powerful superfood—is bursting with nutrients. And it's gaining recognition for its many healing properties and starting to be much more widely available, so nowadays you don't have to go to a sushi restaurant every time you want a bite of sea veggies. And there are many ways to reap their numerous beauty benefits.

Seaweed can be . . .

- **Enjoyed as a delicious part of a meal.** There are many organic products that contain seaweed, and many types of seaweed for you to incorporate into your diet through salads, stir-fries, and smoothies. Chlorella and spirulina are easy to purchase online or in your favorite natural food market, and help to alkalize your body, boost your mood, reduce the free radical damage that can lead to cancer, and regulate thyroid function so you feel beautiful from the inside out. Choose a seaweed salad or miso soup (which contains wakame) at your favorite Japanese restaurant.

- **The new potato chips.** At supermarkets, convenience stores, and even airports, grab a bag of nori—from companies such as GimMe Organic, SeaSnax, or Annie Chun's—filled with an array of nutrients, including vitamins A and C, calcium, and iron.

- **Taken as a supplement.** Schinoussa Sea Greens, my favorite brand of seaweed supplement, offers a potent blend of ethically sourced seaweeds in capsule form.

- **Applied directly to the skin.** As a natural beauty product, seaweed's wealth of essential vitamins, minerals, amino acids, and antioxidants help keep the skin revitalized, moisturized, and youthful, guarding the skin against the harmful effects of environmental pollutants and slowing the aging process. The anti-inflammatory properties in seaweed can also be used to treat skin rashes and wounds. The phytonutrients elevate blood flow and bring a healthy glow to the face. Seaweed wraps detoxify and cleanse the skin by expelling toxins from the pores. Seaweed baths have been used for centuries for their therapeutic effects. The high mineral content of seaweed also helps create healthy, strong, shiny hair.

Our lives become more and more beautiful the more we learn to be kind and care for ourselves.
—**Susan Black**

Beauty Is Authenticity

How ironic is it that an industry that's supposed to be about celebrating beauty has spent the past several decades creating hollow, meaningless images? A true celebration of beauty would never prioritize a shiny, sexy surface over a human being's happiness, health, and connection to nature. The mainstream industry has it backward—our humanity is actually the very source of our beauty.

This understanding of beauty is rapidly taking hold. Through engaging with my two millennial children and their peers, I have witnessed that the old standards are being questioned. As a generation, millennials are moving toward an idea of beauty that has to do with seeing the humanity in everyone.

Many celebrities are leveraging their platforms to redefine the meaning of beauty. Alicia Keys has a particularly inspiring story. Alicia Keys is one celebrity who has actively set aside her makeup regime entirely, describing what, for her, symbolized a mask of inauthenticity: "I was finally uncovering just how much I censored myself, and it scared me. Who was I, anyway? Did I even know HOW to be brutally honest anymore? Who I wanted to be? . . . I found my way to meditation, and I started focusing on clarity and a deeper knowledge of myself. I focused on cultivating strength and conviction and put a practice in place to learn more about the real me."[4]

Alicia still has a daily skin-care regime but takes a simpler, more natural approach, and makes room for regular changes depending on what her skin needs. Sometimes she uses grated cucumber to cool her skin and bring the blood to the surface; sometimes she uses light oils (such as jojoba, hazelnut, or argan); at other times she uses a frozen jade roller to massage her face (jade has been used in Chinese medicine for centuries to help filter toxins and clear the lymphatic system).[5]

I share Alicia's story with you not as a journey I suggest you replicate identically—although, if her holistic beauty regimen intrigues you, it's entirely accessible to anyone. Depending on your personality, it may or may not be authentic for you to forgo makeup altogether. Many people, both women and men, ultimately see makeup as a way to express themselves to the world. In discovering our authentic selves, we have so many options—we just have to discover what makes our inner beauty shine and glow.

When it comes to living authentically, makeup is a topic that can be especially fraught with controversy. But at the end of the day, wearing makeup is just an extension of an entirely natural (and fun) human tendency—to groom ourselves, and to use our external appearance as a physical representation of our true selves. Wearing makeup (and styling our hair, having our nails done, or any other kind of personal grooming) can be powerfully expressive and even artistic.

As Naomi Wolf eloquently stated in *The Beauty Myth*, "She wins who calls herself beautiful and challenges the world to change to truly see her."[6] True to this idea, we feel beautiful when we feel as though we're fully understood, loved, and accepted for exactly who we are. Individuality is the basis for authentic beauty, so it can manifest in countless ways. You might feel most like yourself in no makeup and simple, neutral-colored clothing, or you might feel more comfortable when donning vintage clothes, winged eyeliner, and brightly colored lipstick. But any beauty routine you *do* choose shouldn't be from a place of obligation—it should be an enjoyable, rejuvenating part of your day!

Pause, reflect, and open your heart to your own unique manifestation of a conscious, beautiful lifestyle. Things worth achieving take time, a little experimentation—and honesty. If something isn't working for you, stop and move on. Even if a product is organic, derived from nature, and made with love, it might not be the exact right one for you. When you start implementing a new holistic practice or using a new organic product, ask yourself how it makes you feel. Enjoy this process of self-exploration—I promise it will pay off, and you'll enjoy your connected beauty and radiant health for years to come.

> My vision for the future of beauty is the same one I have always celebrated—the diversity of beauty. Celebrating what the global palette has to offer in terms of skin tones, rituals, ingredients, sisterhood.
> —**Shalini Vadhera**

Beauty Blogs and Podcasts

BEAUTY BLOGS

Kristen Arnett
Organic Beauty Blogger
Organic Beauty Talk
The Beauty Bean
The Clean Beauty Blog

PODCASTS

The Beauty Brains
The Wellness Wonderland

Let Yourself Shine

Beauty begins the moment you decide to be yourself.
—COCO CHANEL

Let me tell you a story that always makes me smile and that helps me connect to what true beauty means. In the early 2000s, Under the Canopy had the opportunity to be part of the *Tyra Banks Show*. We were asked to provide audience members with organic cotton kimonos for what was to be a truly special occasion. The episode was a celebration of womanhood, diversity, and self-acceptance.

Tyra began the show with a bold move. On the count of three she invited the audience to join her in removing their Under the Canopy robes and letting it all hang out. "Freedom! Freedom everyone!" she cried. And they carried on the rest of the show undressed and empowered by body-positive energy. It was truly emotional—Tyra had given the audience permission to be themselves, and created an environment of acceptance and self-love.

At the end of the day, we step into our most radiant beauty when we find freedom, empowerment, authenticity, and happiness. When we're living our truth, connected to who we are, and taking care of our home and ourselves, our inner beauty will *literally* shine through.

How do you express yourself physically and aesthetically? Are you a person who goes for a bold, dramatic, striking look? A soft, flowy, bohemian look? A clean, fresh, barefaced look?

Think about how you're drawn to express yourself through makeup and personal care products. No matter how many, or how few, cosmetics you use, it says something about you. What is the story you're telling? How could that story be even more profound? How could your habits and self-expression feel more authentic, enjoyable, and purposeful?

ECOfy: Beauty Tips

Here are a few of my go-to holistic beauty tips:

- I start and end my day with a ritual—it's not just about the products I use, it's also about self-care. When I wash my face, I use only all-natural/organic cleansers, toners, and moisturizers, and I take the time to minimassage my face with love, which stimulates blood flow in the skin and feels *amazing*. (Pure argan oil—rich in antioxidants and vitamins A and E—is my favorite nighttime skin replenishment.)

- Moisturizing treatments (scrubs and masques) for your skin and hair are incredibly rejuvenating, both emotionally and physically.

- Get enough sleep! And implement self-care and stress management (such as yoga—which, for me, is the ultimate mind-body practice).

- Meditation and breathwork—aside from the fact that they enhance feelings of relaxation and peace, this deep breathing oxygenates the skin and circulates blood to give you that glow.

- Sweat. Whether it's going to a sauna or a steam room, taking a hot yoga class, or going for a long run, sweat is our body's most natural way of detoxing and cleansing.

- Get regular vitamin D, but be sure to protect your skin with a natural sunblock (such as Coola or Badger).

> The defining tenet of the ECOrenaissance is understanding ourselves and each aspect of our lives as essentially and intricately connected to the ecosystems we live in.

This could come in the form of exploring different beauty and personal care products, it could come from starting a regular yoga/breath-work/meditation practice, or getting outside and immersing yourself in nature more often. Personally, I tap into my inner beauty with effortless ease when I'm by the ocean. I'm in my ultimate happy place when I can hear the waves crashing, feel the sun on my skin, and smell the sweet, salty air. In essence, I feel nourished and alive.

We're never separate from the beauty of nature. The defining tenet of the ECOrenaissance is understanding ourselves and each aspect of our lives as essentially and intricately connected to the ecosystems we live in. Nature is the ultimate source of beauty. And when we give ourselves permission to just be, simply as we are, the beauty of the entire universe shines through us. Beauty is timeless because our light is endless.

The DNA of ECOrenaissance Beauty: No Compromise in Function or Quality

- Authentic beauty is within everyone's reach. Connect to your inner being.
- True beauty radiates from the inside out—healthy food, positive attitude, and wellness.
- Food choices impact the overall health of your skin. Eat consciously.
- Beauty regimens can and should include regular self-love and self-care.
- No harmful ingredients such as synthetic fragrances, parabens, phthalates, lead, etc.
- Cruelty-free and no animal testing.
- Less is more.
- Plant-based, organic ingredients, and made with love.
- Share with your friends and family. The more they know, the better off they'll be.
- There are examples of beauty everywhere. Keep your eyes open to the abundance.

Illuminartist Interviews: *Beauty*

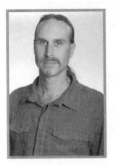

David Bronner, CEO of Dr. Bronner's
www.drbronners.com

Otherwise known as the "cosmic engagement officer" of the top-selling brand of natural soaps in North America and producer of other organic body care and food products, David is one of the world's leading integrity activists and planetary ambassadors.

What is a personal ECOrenaissance tip you can share with readers?

Our daily dietary choices are the most immediate and impactful. Choosing to eat less and better meat, dairy, and eggs from organic, pasture-based farms is crucial, alongside the choice to adopt a more strict plant-based diet.

How did you start your journey toward social purpose?

My granddad Dr. Bronner was an early pioneer in ecological living, and psychedelic experiences after college reinforced the importance of planetary health and survival. We're all One!

Which of the pillars of the ECOrenaissance movement (collaboration, consciousness, community, creativity, connection) resonate most with you and why?

All those principles are important. Picking one, I would say consciousness of the interconnected web of life and the responsibility to care for one another . . . so, actually, community and connection, too.

What is your vision for the future of beauty (and food)?

My vision is that all food we eat and products we consume are based on regenerative organic agriculture, where the farmers and workers involved at both the farm level and postharvest processing are treated fairly. Bam!

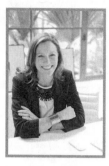

Gregg Renfrew, Founder of Beautycounter

www.beautycounter.com

Gregg's new model marrying conscious business and beauty has become a game-changing win-win for many thousands of people. Check out Beautycounter!

What is a personal ECOrenaissance tip you can share with readers?

Switch every piece of plastic you use to glass. Use filtered water rather than bottled, and turn the lights off when you leave a room. Unplug your electronics. Little things make a big difference if we all do them together.

What is your vision for the future of beauty?

To me, the future of beauty is marked by cleaner products, safer formulas, and significant innovation around natural ingredients—with the customer calling the shots.

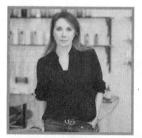

Kiran Stordalen, Cofounder of Intelligent Nutrients (formerly Creative Director of AVEDA)

www.intelligentnutrients.com

Kiran is one of the most beautiful people I know, and her feminine energy and artistic intelligence were added forces behind Horst's brilliant vision at AVEDA. Now running Intelligent Nutrients, Kiran—and Horst's daughter Nicole—have raised the bar on true lasting beauty.

How did you start your journey toward sustainability/social purpose?

Like many idealistic college students, I wanted to do something "meaningful" with my life. I began my career at AVEDA many years ago just as the mission of the company was being cultivated as a platform for environmental and social responsibility, and the importance of our corporate behavior was front and center. The founder of AVEDA, Horst Rechelbacher, was my partner in life and work, and through vision and hard work, and with amazingly talented people, we had the incredible opportunity to create a company that had a sense of purpose greater that the products themselves. Now with Intelligent Nutrients, myself and my business partner, Nicole Rechelbacher, are following in those same footprints, adhering to our heritage with an ever greater and stronger commitment to organic, safe, nontoxic, pure products.

What is your vision for the future of fashion and beauty?

We all want to look and feel our best. I think we're beginning to recognize that going green and looking great are not mutually exclusive. We can create products that make us look and feel beautiful without robbing the world of its beauty. When we pay attention to raw materials, whether it's ingredients, packaging, or textiles, and demonstrate honesty and accountability surrounding those choices—it makes a difference, and that's the future.

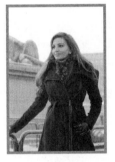

Shalini Vadhera, Founder of Power Beauty Living
www.shalinisworld.com
www.powerbeautyliving.com

Shalini's incredible work has her traveling the world sharing global beauty secrets to transform and inspire. Check out her Passport to Beauty!

What is a personal ECOrenaissance tip you can share with readers?

I've found that one of the best and easiest lifestyle changes that has seemed to have the most impact on the world is kindness. And then using that kindness to pay it forward and help someone who needs it. I have personally seen how it has positively affected the people I have come in contact with and how they have then done the same for others. Seeing that momentum build is amazing.

How did you start your journey toward social purpose?

After launching my first brand, I felt there was a huge void in resources and mentorship for women by women. I launched a women's platform called Power Beauty Living, which has helped women power up their business and their beauty—to have unmatched confidence for unmatched leverage and to balance their lives through tools and techniques that they could do for thirty minutes a day to have a warrior mentality. Every event we have, we partner with a female-focused charity to support and give proceeds to. For my beauty brand, Passport to Beauty, we realized that we really needed to focus on cleaner, safer ingredients as well as sourcing natural ingredients from the global palette.

Which of the pillars of the ECOrenaissance movement (collaboration, consciousness, community, creativity, connection) resonate most with you and why?

They all do, starting with consciousness. You need to be mindful first of the earth, the people, and how you can take a stand for what is right when it comes to protecting our resources as well as supporting the human race. From there, you can build with collaboration, community, creativity, and connection. It's a wonderful thing.

What is your vision for the future of beauty?

My vision for the future of beauty is the same one I have always celebrated—the diversity of beauty. Celebrating what the global palette has to offer in terms of skin tones, rituals, ingredients, sisterhood. Looking at beauty as a holistic approach—inner beauty and how it affects outer beauty. As they say, happy girls are the prettiest girls.

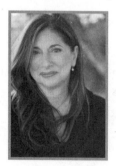

Susan Black, Cofounder of EO Products/Everyone
www.eoproducts.com

One of my favorite women on the planet, Susan is the embodiment of radiant organic beauty on every level. At EO, there's something for Every One.

What is a personal ECOrenaissance tip you can share with readers?

Kindness is vastly underrated. Be kind to yourself and treat everyone the way you would like to be treated. I think kindness is the accessory that enhances every style at every stage of life. Kindness and self-love infuse women with a deep, inherent "femaleness" and a sense of wonder. Our lives become more and more beautiful the more we learn to be kind and care for ourselves. There's this incredible radiance that appears when we love ourselves, and that inner light is the core of what we see as beautiful.

Which of the pillars of the ECOrenaissance movement (collaboration, consciousness, community, creativity, connection) resonate most with you and why?

Can I choose all of the above? Every one of these qualities resonates with me. Here, instead of choosing, I'll make a haiku:

Conscious connection.
Collaborate with others.
Creativity.

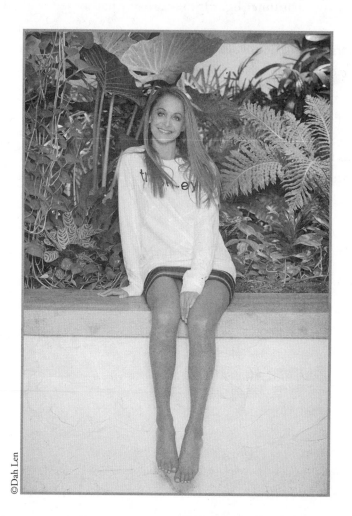

©Dah Len

This photo captures the true meaning of the ECOrenaissance on every level. I'm wearing my much-adored "trash-ey" sweatshirt, cocreated by zero-waste fashion designer Daniel Silverstein, inspired by zero-waste blogger and influencer Lauren Singer, and made from certified organic cotton scraps from my sustainable USA factory, MetaWear. No better place to start my morning than reflecting peacefully in front of this magnificently curated "Plant the Future" crystal-infused garden in the lobby of the eco-fabulous 1 Hotel South Beach.

6

Styling Change

*There is no beauty in the finest cloth if it
makes hunger and unhappiness.*
—GANDHI

Fashion is one of the most powerful forces for transformation in the world. *Why?* People love fashion. We obsess over what's on the runways and what celebrities are wearing. But at an even more basic level, it's something we all relate to. We all wear clothes, and what we choose to dress ourselves in can make a profound statement about our identity, our culture, our values, our aesthetics. We all connect to fashion in our own unique way.

If we look at the history of apparel, it all started with us drawing materials—and inspiration—from nature. But now, fashion has become a commercialized industry that has gotten way out of control—in our globalized economy, the industry functions off of what is essentially slave labor. Cotton farmers are developing a multiplicity of health conditions due to spending long hours in pesticide-drenched fields, and factory workers work up to eighteen hours a day, often in toxic conditions, getting paid next to nothing. And the environmental impact is immense:[1]

- The fashion industry is one of the planet's largest sources of air and water pollution.
- Ten percent of the world's carbon footprint comes from the textile industry.

- Twenty percent of the world's freshwater pollution comes from the textile industry—three trillion gallons of freshwater are being used to treat and dye garments each year.
- Five percent of landfills are filled with textile waste. To give you an idea of what that looks like, in New York City alone, eight million tons of textile scraps go straight from factories into landfills every year.

We've gotten so far away from our connection with the earth, perpetuating a synthetic, toxic, exploitative industry, that it's no longer about our relationship to what we're putting on our bodies as a relationship to ourselves. It's the worst of the worst of the industries if you combine the negative environmental and social effects—but it doesn't have to be that way. The fashion industry has the dual ability to be powerfully transformative or deeply destructive. It all comes down to making empowered, informed decisions. Remember, the worlds of style and sustainability are not mutually exclusive. You don't have to give up anything. In fact, you get *more* when you choose conscious fashion.

> The fashion industry has the dual ability to be powerfully transformative or deeply destructive. It all comes down to making empowered, informed decisions.

For the most part, people just don't buy clothing that's uncomfortable or unflattering, no matter how eco-friendly it might be. First and foremost, clothes need to be stylish, soft, and of high quality. Fashion brands are starting to sell sustainable apparel on the premise that it's just great apparel—and *oh, by the way*, it also happens to be ethical and eco-friendly. The ECOrenaissance movement is not about making fashion sustainable; it's about making sustainability fashionable.

> The ECOrenaissance movement is not about making fashion sustainable; it's about making sustainability fashionable.

In this chapter, I'll guide you along my journey into the wonderful world of sustainable fashion. We'll explore the environmental and humanitarian consequences of "fast fashion"; look at new, inventive, eco-chic models; and outline ways you can join this rapidly growing movement.

My Journey into ECOfashion

In the early 1990s, I was already well on my way to promoting conscious living, consuming a macrobiotic diet and beginning Gulliver's Living & Learning Center (which later became the Institute for Integrative Nutrition). I didn't know it at the time, but my involvement in healthy and organic food would pave the way for me to discover the world of ECOfashion, which was, at that time, almost entirely untapped. Through mutual acquaintances, I had the pleasure of meeting with the founder of Deja Shoes, a progressive, innovative company that created shoes from recycled rubber tires. Her story moved me, and a lightbulb went off. I thought *wow, conscious fashion*. We had already opened an AVEDA salon in the school, and I started to connect the dots from food to beauty. It was suddenly clear that fashion was the most natural next step.

At about the same time, I had developed a relationship with the Rodale Institute, an independent research and agricultural learning facility developed in the 1970s and responsible for coining the term "organic." I had been introduced to Anthony Rodale at the Natural Products Expo, which was the beginning of a lifelong friendship. He shared with me some work he was doing at the institute on the impact of cotton farming, which opened my mind irreversibly.

I had been wearing cotton and using it in bedding my whole life, and was always drawn more to natural fibers for their breathability. Like many of us, I assumed cotton was a safe choice because it's a natural fiber. I had no idea what went into farming cotton using the conventional method. Anthony and I started to connect dots as I learned that 60 percent of cotton was going into the food stream in bread products, oils, and seed as the primary ingredient in cow feed. There is an inextricable connection between food and fiber in agriculture. You can't really support organic food without supporting organic cotton, because they're often growing side by side, and the methodology is the same.

Intrigued and wanting to learn more, I decided to dive deeper into my exploration of the cotton industry.

- **Working conditions:** I found, to my horror, that most of the world's cotton farmers live and work in destitute, appalling conditions. There is an increasing lack of attention to farmer welfare, especially in regard to awareness around cotton pesticides. Most farmers around the world live in dire poverty and are illiterate. They get lured in by seed companies to use pesticides that are ultimately harmful to their health, and they don't understand what they're getting into. They don't have the resources to defend themselves, ask questions, or demand better conditions. They're victims of an industry that's destructive to their health and the health of their families—respiratory conditions, skin issues, and even cancer are rampant in conventional cotton farming areas.

- **The pesticide treadmill:** Less than 3 percent of the world's agriculture is cotton, yet almost 20 percent of the world's most harmful insecticides, and nearly 10 percent of the most toxic pesticides, are used in the cotton industry, making it *the most* pesticide-intensive crop grown on the planet.[2] The pesticides used by farmers not only kill cotton pests but also decimate populations of beneficial insects such as ladybugs and parasitic wasps. Because their natural enemies have been eradicated, these target insects, which were once only minor nuisances for farmers, become greater problems, and ever-increasing quantities of toxic chemicals must be sprayed to keep them in check. The insects also build resistance to pesticides, so farmers become stuck in an endless cycle known as the "pesticide treadmill"—forced to pay high prices for the toxic chemicals their genetically modified seeds require, and forced to administer these chemicals with little to no means of protection. They go into total despair as their health becomes compromised, bugs get out of control, and they're forced to leverage their farms. In India, every half hour a conventional cotton farmer commits suicide—by drinking pesticides.

  Farmers in the United States apply more than a quarter of a pound of chemical fertilizers and pesticides for every pound of cotton harvested. When the herbicide Roundup was invented, those numbers started to artificially drop, but currently they're going way back up. When all nineteen cotton-growing stages are tallied, cotton crops account for nearly 25 percent of all the pesticides used in the United States. Some of these chemicals are among the most toxic classified by the US Environmental Protection Agency.[3] In developing countries, where regulations are less stringent, the amount of herbicides and insecticides, and their toxicity, are often far greater than in the United States.

As a result, the World Health Organization estimates that at least three million people are poisoned by pesticides, with twenty thousand unintentional deaths a year; 99 percent of fatalities are from developing countries.[4]

- **Child labor and pesticides:** Despite being particularly vulnerable to poisoning, child laborers throughout the world risk exposure to hazardous pesticides through participation in cotton production. In India and Uzbekistan, children are directly involved in cotton pesticide application, while in Pakistan, Egypt, and Central Asia, child laborers work in cotton fields either during or following the spraying season. Children are also often the first victims of pesticide poisonings, even if they don't participate in spraying, due to the proximity of their homes to cotton fields, the reuse of empty pesticide containers, or the widespread contamination of drinking water sources. Most conventional cotton farmers are women, who are even walking through the fields with babies in slings and pesticide tanks on their backs. This is outrageous. And they have no idea until it's too late.

  The results for agrarian communities in Southeast Asia have been particularly devastating. Children are suffering from severe deformities and developmental delays; individuals of all ages are being diagnosed with many forms of cancer. Yet their economic vulnerability forces them back to work. It's important to understand that the rate at which we consume new clothes made of conventional cotton in the First World also forces these communities back to a highly toxic work environment. Cotton represents more than a third of the world's fiber use.

Needless to say, going down the rabbit hole of cotton farming got me thinking about the importance of organic fibers, and the impact of style in general. When I first started, I used to ask this question: *Is there any reason why I can't create the same garments that exist in the market, only substituting organic cotton?* And what I learned was that, just as in the case of food, organic products are even better.

I wanted to translate everything I had learned through food into my fashion ventures. In the words of Jerome Irving Rodale, founder of the Rodale Institute, "Organic is not a fad. It has been a long-established practice—much more firmly grounded than the current chemical flair. Present agricultural practices are leading us downhill."[5]

The same can be said of fast fashion practices as a whole. Retailers such as Zara and Forever 21 are spitting out new collections every week—a far cry from the industry's traditional four seasons per year. The world now consumes a staggering eighty billion garments per year (three-quarters of which end up in our landfills)—up 400 percent from just two decades ago. (Check out Lucy Siegle's book *To Die For: Is Fashion Wearing Out the World?*.)

The systems currently in place simply aren't working. We need to overhaul the methods used in fashion related to agriculture and mass scale manufacturing to show a greater respect for the people and the planetary resources involved. One in six people work in the global fashion industry, with a majority of these workers (mostly women) earning less than three dollars a day. As J. I. Rodale says, the "current chemical flair" isn't better in the long run than the way farming has occurred naturally for millennia. In addition to the financial exploitation of these farmers, hundreds of thousands have killed themselves as a result of going into debt to buy chemically dependent, genetically modified seeds.

Cotton: A Natural Product?

Many people I've spoken to assume cotton is organic or environmentally friendly because it's grown in nature. And though it's true that cotton is grown in nature, it's usually:

- heavily sprayed with pesticides and herbicides,
- bleached with chlorine, and
- processed with toxic chemicals such as formaldehyde and ammonia, as well as heavy metals.

At the end of the day, the perception of cotton as "all natural" is the result of manipulative marketing strategies. I often compare cotton to milk, because people have thought for so long that "milk is natural," but when we pull back the curtain on dairy, the exploitative, unhealthy, wasteful practices of the industry are self-evident.

The cotton industry is not so different. And to add to the environmental degradation and human exploitation perpetuated by the industry, conventional cotton can actually be harmful to individual health. Pesticides, synthetic dyes, formaldehyde, chlorine bleach, heavy metals, and brighteners can get absorbed through the skin—our largest organ for absorption (as outlined in chapter 5, on beauty). There are more than eight thousand synthetic chemicals used in the textile industry, many of which are harmful and added to cotton garments. And cotton can be on our skin 24-7, via T-shirts, jeans, and other clothing, as well as in items such as bedsheets, bathrobes, and towels.

In contrast, certified organic cotton—specifically Global Organic Textile Standard (GOTS) certified—is grown GMO-free, is never treated with fungicides, synthetic pesticides, or fertilizers, and according to PE International and the Textile Exchange, uses 71 percent less water and 62 percent less energy than conventionally produced cotton. If a product is GOTS certified, it's also free of heavy metals, chlorine bleach, formaldehyde, and aromatic solvents, making it free of carcinogens and other toxic chemicals, as well as many allergens. (For more information on organic cotton, check out aboutorganiccotton.org.)

When I was first starting out in fashion, I instantly realized the enormous potential of fashion to be a major catalyst for change, in terms of closing the loop, promoting a circular economy and soil health, and minimizing chemical and energy use, waste, and water pollution. But I always knew that it would be impossible to sell fashion to the majority of people based solely on the fact of it being sustainable, organic, regenerative, zero waste, or Fair Trade. So I made it my mission to do away with the existing stigmas around sustainability in fashion. I had observed three main misconceptions:

1. Style and sustainability were mutually exclusive.
2. It would be too expensive.
3. People were suspicious about labeling: "How can I tell if it's really organic, ethically made, and/or free of harmful chemicals?"

I set about addressing these three stigmas, and I found that it was much simpler and more intuitive than I had been led to believe.

> Shop at small businesses, shop locally produced
> goods. Know and wear your impact.
> **—Rosario Dawson and Abrima Erwiah**

Making Sustainability Stylish

Because of my business background, I understand that how you package things can make all the difference in the world in how they're received. People are always initially drawn to the surface, to the way things look. So a beautiful, elegant style can present an essential means of planting a seed of consciousness, one that the consumer may not even be aware of at first. Horst had mastered that concept in his brilliant, beautiful design for AVEDA. He was genius in his aesthetic discipline and in the way he brought products to life. I made it my goal to harness this same concept in fashion. One example of this idea stands out particularly clearly in my memory.

In the early days of Under the Canopy, I created a garment in collaboration with my dear friend Romio Shrestha. Romio had just released a book titled *Celestial Gallery*, a large-format art tome featuring striking Tibetan-style mandala paintings of the great Buddha and related teachings. I was particularly drawn to an image of the seven chakras, or spiritual energy centers in the body, which Romio let me borrow and adapt on an organic cotton tank top. We chose to highlight the three highest chakra points—representing expression, intuition, and emotion—via Sanskrit embroidery or appliqué, and it was a total hit. People really loved this tank.

> People are always initially drawn to the surface, to the way things look. So a beautiful, elegant style can present an essential means of planting a seed of consciousness.

What stuck with me was that people who didn't know about chakras were drawn to this beautifully designed tank top and still loved it as much as those who were aware of the fact that those chakras represent your highest level of divinity. We had planted a seed of knowledge through the garment, which ended up prompting many to discover the wisdom of the chakras, and how they regulate our life force energy by absorbing and holding memory and vibration. The tank, a statement piece unto itself, was a real conversation starter. I loved hearing the many stories customers shared about their experience wearing it, and how interest and awareness around the chakras continued to grow with each wear.

Cutting Unnecessary Costs

The second stigma to be addressed was the concept that sustainable, ethical apparel was much too pricey. Green fashion, in the early years, was very aspirational, but it wasn't accessible. It was limited to high-fashion models on runways; as a result, it ended up being either too out-there or too expensive. But I learned that by navigating supply chains efficiently, and cutting out markups and middlemen (generally there can be seven to ten levels in a supply chain, with each step of the way taking a markup), I've been able to add value and retain competitive prices. The fact that I actually knew the people in my entire holistic supply chain—the farmers, spinners, knitters, sewers, and finishers—was absolutely unheard of at the time.

> You don't have to be wealthy to buy sustainably, you just have to know where to go to get it.

From farm to finished fashion, I re-created the fashion supply chain, and people thought I was a little crazy. But now, everyone from Hanky Panky to Kering to H&M and Target is launching organic and sustainable wares. You don't have to be wealthy to buy sustainably, you just have to know where to go to get it (refer to the list of ECOfashion companies below for guidance).

Radical Transparency

The last stigma to be addressed was the issue of transparency, and ensuring that consumers could be secure in their purchase of organic cotton and/or eco-friendly apparel. I was on the small team in the 1990s that wrote the very first organic textile certification for the United States. And we soon discovered that because textiles cross boundaries and borders every day, the only way to assure full global traceability was to create an international certification. So we collaborated with other trade associations from the United Kingdom, Germany, and Japan, and developed what is known today as the Global Organic Textile Standard (GOTS). This is the premium and platinum standard for farm to finished product certified organic textiles.

There is now labeling to help us avoid supporting companies that treat their garments with toxic chemicals. Look for GOTS, OEKO-TEX, and Cradle to Cradle certified products. In addition, the Textile Exchange has animal welfare certifications for responsible wool, down, and leather, too.

As shared in my interview on Gwyneth Paltrow's Goop.com, what chemicals should we be most worried about in our apparel and home textiles?[6]

CHEMICAL	USED FOR	FOUND IN	CONCERNS
GLYPHOSATE	Herbicide in cotton growing	Cotton textiles	Carcinogenic; potentially linked to autism
CHLORINE BLEACH	Whitening and stain removal	Natural fiber/cotton processing (such as denim)	Asthma and respiratory problems
FORMALDEHYDE	Mainly used for wrinkle-free; also shrinkage; carrier for dyes/prints	Natural fabrics such as cotton, or anything that's been dyed or printed	Carcinogenic
VOCs	Solvents used in all parts of the textile supply chain, particularly for printing	Finished textiles, especially printed (natural and synthetic)	Off-gassing, which is a huge issue for workers. VOCs cause developmental and reproductive system damage, skin/eye irritation, and liver and respiratory problems. Some VOCs are carcinogens.
PFCs	Creating durable water resistance; as stain repellant/manager	Finished textiles, especially printed (natural and synthetic, especially uniforms and outdoor clothing)	Carcinogenic, bioaccumulative (builds up in bloodstream), persistent, and toxic in the environment

CHEMICAL	USED FOR	FOUND IN	CONCERNS
BROMINATED FLAME RETARDANTS	Used to stop clothes from burning	Required on children's clothing	Neurotoxins, endocrine disruptors, carcinogens, bioaccumulative
AMMONIA	Provides shrink resistance	Natural fabrics	Absorbed into lungs; can burn eye, nose, throat
HEAVY METALS (LEAD, CHROMIUM VI, CADMIUM, ANTIMONY, ETC.)	For dyeing; chromium VI is used in leather tanning, and antimony is used to make polyester	Finished textiles, especially dyed and/or printed (natural and synthetic)	Highly toxic; can cause DNA/reproductive issues, damage blood cells, kidney, liver; environmental damage
PHTHALATES/ PLASTISOL	Used in printing	Printing inks/processes	Endocrine disruptors

Data from Greenpeace Detox Campaign,[7] European Chemicals Agency,[8] and Chemical Safety Facts.[9]

Transparent companies will make their practices very clear on their websites. Some examples of these mission-driven, nontoxic, ethical brands include Stella McCartney, Outerknown, Patagonia, Mara Hoffman, Reformation, Eileen Fisher, Prana, and Coyuchi. Most of these brands will only use certified organic cotton in their cotton products. In addition to being at 94 percent organic cotton, Eileen Fisher is also making 20 percent of their products in America.

Commitment to Change

According to the Textile Exchange, some encouraging positive commitments, as of 2017, include:[10]

- More than thirty-six major brands have pledged to achieve 100 percent sustainable cotton by 2025, including four on *Forbes* magazine's list of the world's ten largest global apparel brands and three of the top UK clothing retailers. This initiative—with brands such as Nike, Adidas, Burberry, Timberland, H&M, and IKEA, to name just a few—is being driven by the Prince of Wales and organized by the prince's International Sustainability Unit (ISU), in collaboration with Marks & Spencer and the Soil Association (UK), to facilitate consensus on solving the world's most pressing environmental challenges.

- The fashion and textile industries are adopting a growing amount of preferred, more sustainable fibers and practices. Recycled polyester usage grew by 58 percent, and more than forty renowned textile, apparel, and retail companies have committed to increasing their use by at least 25 percent by 2020.

- Global Fashion Agenda announced that 64 companies representing 143 brands and a combined value of no less than 7.5 percent of the global fashion market—including C&A, Inditex, Kering, H&M, Target, Tommy Hilfiger, and VF Corp—signed a commitment to accelerate the transition to a circular fashion system.

The use of leather for fashion has a massive environmental impact. Massive. From unnecessary water consumption to high emissions of greenhouse gases and polluting chemicals. So for me it's really about questioning the process.

—**Stella McCartney**

Cultivating Personal Style

Looking back, I realize how organically my story all fell together. From a young age, I've always been very attracted to fashion and aesthetics—it's funny how shades of our childhood identities remain present in our adult lives. In my senior year of high school, my dear friend Eric Rutherford (@mr.rutherford) and I were voted best dressed in our class. Die-hard Madonna fans, art aficionados, and creatives marching to the beat of our own drums, Eric and I both loved to act, sing, dance, draw, travel, and embrace our expressive, artistic selves. When we met at age twelve, we were drawn to each other, deeply and intuitively connecting—and we retain that connection to this day. We still call each other wonder-twin. Whenever we were together, we felt the power of cocreation.

ECOfy: Fashion Faves

Here are a few curated websites, and fashion or accessory brands I recommend:

Able Made	Joanne Stone	Modavanti	SITO (by Mercola
Alternative Apparel	Jewelry	MUD Jeans	.com)
Bead & Reel	Kaight	Nalu	SkunkFunk
Behno	LIVARI	Outerknown	SOKO Jewelry
CHNGE	Lux & Eco	PACT	Stella McCartney
Coyuchi	Made in Earth	People Tree	SVILU
EDUN	Jewelry	Reformation	Triarchy Denim
Eileen Fisher	Maison de	Rent the Runway	Under the Canopy
Farm to Home	Mode ·	Reve en Vert	Warby Parker
Groceries Apparel	Maiyet	Satya Jewelry	Zero Waste Daniel
Hanky Panky	Mara Hoffman	Shop Ethica	(ZWD)
Indigenous	MetaWear	Shop Helpsy	

And for your outdoor and performance wear, shop Prana and Patagonia.

Fast-forward thirty-eight short years, and we're both in the fashion industry, curating creative consciousness and lasting change through the lens of authenticity and beautiful design. Eric is now a highly successful model, and has cultivated an incredible existence. Eternally connected, we embraced the ECOrenaissance lifestyle together from a very young age, determined to live our truths in an unstoppable way. While Surya was a mentor, Eric was like my male counterpart. We both had such a strong sense of individuality, and this manifested both in our creative fashion choices and progressive lifestyles.

I share this with you to emphasize how much style is at the core of how we express ourselves. Personal style is the externalization of your internal voice, the first impression you give others about your ideas and passions, your sense of self, your identity. And you can tell so much about a person when you meet them by the way they carry themselves, through their style. Unique style makes me smile. I'm so drawn to the brave souls who aren't living their life under the guise of what they're "supposed" to be doing, and who are emanating a sense of individuality and confidence.

To green your wardrobe and cultivate a beautiful, unique style:

- Instead of buying three fast fashion shirts, buy one high-quality, ethical piece that costs more but will last you forever and will become a staple of your wardrobe.
- Support local designers and locally made clothes.
- Shop vintage or thrift for unique items and to reduce the consumption of new materials. Vintage clothing is an especially good choice, as typically, older clothing is not as toxic as clothing being made today.
- When buying new, purchase from responsible brands and retailers that are committed to supply chain transparency and traceability.
- Repurpose clothing—or, if you're crafty, design and sew your own. There is no better way to cultivate a unique wardrobe while saving the planet.
- Rent your casual, work, travel, and/or dressy attire from companies such as MUD Jeans or Rent the Runway.

We want our style to represent who we are at the core, to align with our true selves, to tell a story that resonates. Imagine if each piece of clothing we wore *actually* told a story. With the majority of today's fashion, most of us would be telling a story of worker abuse and toxic chemical use. Instead, what if we could transform our choices so much that every story we told was a positive one? What if, when asked about what we're wearing, we could proudly say that our clothing choices are supporting women in rural areas who are breaking the cycle of poverty and disease and are starting their own companies, using sustainable agriculture to create beautiful, healthy textiles? Each of us has the power to support these positive changes, these transformative stories.

In my own life, I always seek out not just the *what* but also the *why*. And then it's all about the *how*. I want my clothes to tell a story that I'm proud of and excited about. I can't wait for people to ask me what I'm wearing. I even get excited when people are in my apartment and compliment my throw pillows, and I can tell them how they're certified organic—grown and sewn ethically in India.

The whole premise of the ECOrenaissance is tuning back in to our own truths. The only way we can connect to those is to let go of all the layers of what we've been taught and told and trust our gut. We choose whether to be leaders or followers in our style choices. When we look at many style icons, they're making statements that transcend the trends of their time. Oftentimes a shift in what's acceptable or fashionable occurs simply because one person was brave enough to try something new—or project a new meaning—taking something familiar, even mundane, and framing it in a novel way.

When people copy celebrities' style, what they're *really* copying is the glowing strength, self-confidence, and individuality emitted by people who are unapologetically living their truth. It's not necessarily about the aesthetics; it's more about the personality. There is ritual or ceremony in getting dressed. We *become*; we *transform*.

It's intuitive that people connect what they put on their body to how they're acting. That's the way we're wired. But something that's even more powerful is *authenticity*—when we add consciousness and purpose to our choices. We can feel completely different when we wear a product that we're proud to be wearing. Fashion can be a catalyst to transform, ignite, and activate. It has such a deep influence on the way we interact with the world. We become our best selves, connected from the outside in, radiant from the inside out, and strengthened by our authenticity. There's no one style that works for everyone. Feeling empowered through fashion comes as a natural next step to selecting clothing that makes you feel comfortable, confident, and delighted.

Something that's even more powerful is *authenticity*—when we add consciousness and purpose to our choices. We can feel completely different when we wear a product that we're proud to be wearing.

Cultivating Authentic Style

In terms of my own style, I have broad tastes, and as a result, an eclectic closet to show for it. Fashion has always been a place of endless opportunity and inspiration for me, a place where I'm free to reinvent myself and enhance different aspects of my character. I love to play around and try new things. I've never felt the need to dress like everyone else. I have always felt free to think for myself and to change my mind—never a slave to fashion trends. It feels very natural to me for style to change and evolve, as style is guided from a fluid place within us and influenced by the diversity around us. But throughout these shifts and changes, I have always felt a responsibility to understand and then consider the relationship between the clothes I wear and how they impact the world around me.

I gravitate toward conscious, comfortable, warm, sensual, sexy outfits that feel beautiful on my skin. In search of new styles, I like to travel off the beaten path, to boutiques with a really curated feel, and to vintage stores where I can hunt for truly unique and quality pieces. I have learned to tap into my soul when I try something on and ask myself at a gut level, "How do I feel in this?" and "What story is this telling?" Not just, "How does this look on me?" I encourage you to nurture your internal style compass in this way. Step away from the mirror and be present. Sit. Stand. Move around. Focus on your own perspective from within the outfit, as opposed to how you imagine others will see you. When we dress for ourselves, we enjoy a state of stylistic freedom.

The Green Carpet Challenge

On the red carpet, the question is always, "What are you wearing?" Imagine if the answer wasn't just another high-end designer, but someone truly groundbreaking such as Daniel Silverstein of Zero Waste Daniel (www.zerowastedaniel.com), who collects scraps from domestic factories and sorts them by color, then creates beautiful, zero-waste designs. His clothes are not only cutting down on needless waste, but also solving a huge waste issue within the textile industry. He's part of the solution, and he's also making beautiful, unique designs in the process.

The Green Carpet movement is challenging celebrities to show their support for green fashion. It was started by Livia Firth, who wanted to "use the fact that I was going to be walking those red carpets next to Colin [Firth] to campaign about environmental and social justice issues through my gown."[11] It started as a personal challenge in 2010, but it has grown exponentially, embraced by high-fashion companies such as Stella McCartney, Gucci, Net-A-Porter, and Sergio Rossi (to name a few) and represented by celebrities such as Penelope Cruz, Keira Knightley, Emma Watson, Lupita Nyong'o, Margot Robbie, and more. The GCC awards a brandmark to any company that aligns with their ten principles, which are:

1. Transparency
2. No child labor
3. Fair work
4. Community
5. Traceability
6. Preservation of resources and environment

7. Recycle and reuse
8. Pollution minimization
9. Resource management
10. Animal welfare

The Changing Tides of Fashion

**Fashion is not something that exists in dresses only.
Fashion is in the sky, in the street, fashion has to do
with ideas, the way we live, what is happening.**

—COCO CHANEL

Fashion is a reflection of style, of what's happening within culture. Compared to style, fashion is more about the collective. It has to do with trends, with eras, with movements, whereas style has to do with the individual. Fashion is more about what people are defining as "in" at any given moment, and can often become all about following trends. Style, on the other hand, is more about personal expression. Style represents individual choice, and fashion can be bought. When I coined the term "ECOfashion," I thought of it as a play on ideas about fashion—I wanted to redefine and revolutionize the parameters of the industry.

Currently, we're bombarded with options when it comes to fashion. In the past, fashion seasons existed on a literally *seasonal* basis, and clothing styles would change with the weather. Now a fashion season lasts just weeks. This construct is not accidental—trends cycle through at such a rapid pace for the sole purpose of persuading consumers to buy more. As a result, it's easy to get stuck in the cycle of paying ever lower prices for trendy clothes (without questioning how, exactly, those prices could possibly be so low), and then quickly abandoning them in favor of next season's influx of equally short-lived trends.

But even as fast fashion becomes more out of control, hurtling toward its breaking point, we're becoming more and more free to overcome the herd mentality of fashion and move toward defining our own core style that resonates with who we truly are. Suppose you endeavor to live a sustainable life and be a conscious consumer. If you haven't already, you might consider gravitating to an individual style that's more connected to brands that minimize their impact on human and planetary health.

We learn so much about who people are by virtue of the strong style statement they're making. Now more than ever, authenticity is becoming so paramount in today's popular culture, and we're no longer blinded by the mob mentality of what's "in." We have a tremendous opportunity to dress with purpose, by choosing brands that are supporting our planet's ecosystems and very existence. People are making a new kind of fashion statement, one that's in sync with who we are at a deeper level. Fashion is fun, and it's okay to take inspiration from it—but don't get boxed in. Go deeper, by defining your own unique style, in a way that represents who you are in every way.

Stop and reflect on some of these questions before purchasing:

- How many times will I wear this?
- Who made this? Is it a green or conscious brand?
- What is it made out of? Are the materials safe?
- Does my purchase support a company that supports the world?
- Do I have something similar, or is this piece unique?
- Do I *love* this piece, or could I do without it?
- What do I plan to do with the clothes this item might replace?
- What about it speaks to me? What story does it tell?

The me-me-me mind-set of fashion has trickled all the way down from the top of the supply chain to the consumer level, without any thought to the consequences. Fast fashion is completely out of control. We have to slow down. We have to think about buying less, buying smart. Here are some suggestions:

- Invest in higher-quality garments that give good value over time.
- Select garments you truly love, as they will prove to be timeless wardrobe staples.
- Adopt Livia Firth's "thirty wears" rule: only purchase what you're sure you'll wear a minimum of thirty times.

- Can't commit to thirty wears? Or maybe you're shopping for a specific event and know you'll wear it only once? Tap into the steadily growing sharing culture, and rent designer wares on a weekly or monthly basis. Outlets such as Rent-Frock-Repeat, Rent the Runway, or Bag Borrow or Steal provide haute styles at a fraction of the cost and environmental impact.

So many people are waking up, and we need to support the companies that are conscious and driving change. We also need to encourage the companies that aren't embracing more mindful practices to start getting on board. When we vote with our dollars, we're part of a powerful collective demand for change (which we will discuss more in chapter 7).

This shift is happening because people can no longer tune out the readily available information exposing the destructive, exploitative practices of the fashion industry. In our ability to pull the curtain back, the Internet has afforded us an abundance of clarity when it comes to the impact of fashion. Even though sustainable, ethical fashion is still an industry in its infancy, awareness is growing, and better choices are becoming more and more available and affordable.

Now we have the amazing opportunity to ensure that what we wear is in resonance with who we are and supports our values at a deeper level. It's invigorating. It's fun. It takes fashion to a whole new level, physically and spiritually. We have the power to look good, feel good, and do good in the world, all at once. Collectively, we just have to design this reality. And we *can*, because we've essentially designed everything that exists. We can *re-create* and *cocreate*. This is the rebirth, the ECOrenaissance.

> We have the power to look good, feel good, and do good in the world, all at once. Collectively, we just have to design this reality.

Baby Steps

In making the shift in your own lifestyle and wardrobe, it's all about baby steps. You don't have to throw out your whole closet, or even stop shopping at your favorite stores, but choose wisely. Notice the retailers and brands that you're already supporting, whether or not they're moving in this direction. You don't necessarily have to abandon what you're comfortable with, but don't limit yourself. Open a new door.

- If you're a Target or an H&M fan, begin browsing their conscious collections.

- Did you know there's Under the Canopy organic bedding online at Macy's and Bed, Bath and Beyond and Farm to Home organic textiles at Thrive Market and possibly soon on QVC? Check these out; you might look at organic textiles differently. And then when it comes in the mail and you put it on your bed, you might sleep better, knowing that both the source and the story are so positive.

- To take it one step further, seek out the companies that are embracing the movement and taking action as part of the solution. You can see this change in every category and at every price point. Seek clothing made from organic fibers, recycled, upcycled, or dead-stock materials, or that utilize a zero-waste design model, such as the Zero Waste Daniel line.

Creativity is about finding ways around obstacles, rethinking things, being creative within every moment of change.

—**Mara Hoffman**

Driving Fashion Forward

We're in a true fashion revolution, and each of us can play a part in *styling change* for a better world. So what else can we do to harness the power of fashion as a force for change and positivity?

Considering the seventeen sustainable development goals put forth by the United Nations is a good place to start. On the first of January 2016, world leaders adopted seventeen tenets of the 2030 Agenda for Sustainable Development in historic unanimity. These are:[12]

1. No poverty
2. No hunger

3. Good health and well-being
4. Quality education
5. Gender equality
6. Clean water and sanitation
7. Affordable and clean energy
8. Decent work and economic growth
9. Industry, innovation, and infrastructure
10. Reduced inequalities
11. Sustainable cities and communities
12. Responsible consumption and production
13. Climate action
14. Life below water
15. Life on land
16. Peace, justice, and strong institutions
17. Partnerships for the goals

Over the next twelve years, countries will mobilize efforts to end all forms of poverty, fight inequalities, and tackle climate change, while ensuring that no one is left behind. Businesses will be powerful in driving this change, no matter what happens at the governmental level. The train is leaving the station, and businesses have been activated. It may or may not be in parallel with government. But at this point, business is more powerful than government to drive this kind of change. We will discuss this more in chapter 7.

Within the fashion industry, there exist both urgent needs and real opportunities to address these actions. The United Nations' tenet five, gender equality, is of particular significance. The garment industry is and has historically been one of the most female-dominated industries in the world. Today more than 70 percent of garment workers in China are women; in Bangladesh, 85 percent; and in Cambodia, women represent up to 90 percent of the fashion workforce.[13]

ECOfy: Online Resources

Some of the best resources for engaging with this ECOfabulous lifestyle are not much different from other magazines and blogs you may already be following. Include these blogs and online publications in your regular browsing material:

AWEAR World
ECOcult.com
EcoSalon.com
EcoWarriorPrincess.net
Fashionheroes.eco
FashionmeGreen.com
FashionPositive.org
FashionRevolution.org
FashionTakesAction.com
Magnifeco.com
Remake.world
Sustainably-chic.com

"Fashion is a feminist issue," says fellow ECOfashion pioneer Safia Minney, founder of World Fair Trade Day and the clothing line People Tree, the first ever to be awarded the World Fair Trade Organization Fair Trade product label. "Fashion companies are trading faster, harder and using the lack of legislation, transparency, consumer awareness, and a growing unskilled population of young women in the developing world" to their advantage.[14]

Here in the West, we continue to battle lingering discrepancies in equal opportunities for women in the workplace. You can imagine that the dynamic in the developing countries where our fashion is made is even further behind. Higher-skilled and higher-paid roles such as cutting are usually performed by men. Management positions almost exclusively go to men. What's more, export factories tend to hire young women before they're married or become pregnant, and let them go once they are. Childcare is not accessible, and to work, mothers are often forced to leave children with extended family a great distance away.

The Bangladesh Rana Plaza factory collapse in April 2013 was a pivotal moment for an industry that's long been squeezing maximum output from humble, unregulated operations. The world looked on as more and more bodies were dragged from the rubble of the eight-story building containing five garment factories, which was structurally unfit to house heavy, vibrating industrial sewing machinery along with thousands of employees. In the days leading up to the collapse, workers reported cracks in the walls of the building. Many fled from fear, but most were bribed back to work, threatened with the loss of wages. More than 1,133 workers perished in the tragedy, and thousands more were left to cope with injuries and permanent impairments. Hundreds were never found, and remain in the rubble to this day; 80 percent of the employees at Rana Plaza were women between the ages of eighteen and twenty.[15]

Empowering Women, Seeking Solutions

One of my favorite business models is a co-op called Chetna Organic, which provides microfinance loans to female farmers. These women are now creating thriving secondary businesses. And what started as a small handful of cotton farmers now encompasses over thirty-five thousand farmers and countless small businesses; it's an amazing example of a flourishing business model whose upward growth is directly correlated to its capacity for social change. Learn more at www.chetnaorganic.org.

Many familiar Western fashion brands were implicated in the collapse, but what's maybe more important to acknowledge is the complete ubiquity of this business model, and the identical circumstances that exist right now in unregulated factories in other vulnerable countries. What's equally critical to note is that this devastating loss was completely preventable.

At this stage in the movement, few leaders have shown the conviction and commitment of Livia Firth, editor at *Vogue UK*, and founder of ECOAge Consulting and the Green Carpet Challenge. The film she produced with director Andrew Morgan, *The True Cost*, presents a great overview of the challenges the industry faces, as well as the fallout from Rana Plaza. In collaboration with the Lawyers' Circle, TrustLaw, and the Clean Clothes Campaign, Livia is working on a new legal study on global wages, which will build evidence to support the now widely recognized need for an international living wage. This standard will help to address the exploitation and slavery still rife in the fashion sector, arguing that a living wage is a fundamental human right, and as such, the duty of both companies and governments to uphold.

Other Fashion Documentaries to Check Out
River Blue
Driving Fashion Forward with Amber Valletta
Thread Documentary (still a work in progress)

> It's about putting people and the planet first. It's simple gestures like asking yourself: Who made my clothes? Who participated in the making of my clothes?
> —**Rosario Dawson and Abrima Erwiah**

Who Made My Clothes?

Across the world this game-changing question has marked a crusade that only continues to grow. Since 2013, April 24 has been known as Fashion Revolution Day, part of a global movement committed to transparency within the industry and that mobilizes individuals such as you and me to ask about the brands we wear, "Who made my clothes?"—a simple yet powerful inquiry that's much harder to answer than it should be. As manufacturing contracts are outsourced and undercut and outsourced again to generate the most profit for the lowest investment, many big brands completely lose track of where materials are coming from, who their contractors really are, and where the work is being done.

In 2017, from nearly one hundred countries around the world, hundreds of thousands of people took part in Fashion Revolution Week, connected on social media by the hashtag #whomademyclothes. Be sure to check out www.fashionrevolution.org and join the movement. Attend your local events on April 24 (and often throughout the week), or be bold and start something in your community.

Other ECOfashion campaigns to watch:

Beyond the Label
Canopy Planet
Greenpeace Detox Fashion
NRDC Clean Clothes
Redress
Regeneration International's "Care What You Wear"

I suggest thinking about one alternative that helps to reduce a single-use item in your life, something easy, and then commit to it.
—Lauren Singer

Take Action!

It's important to remember our own role as consumers in driving positive change. In addition to the enormous impact of manufacturing clothes, the most environmentally damaging phase in a garment's life cycle occurs after we have acquired the garment, in the "postconsumer use phase," which essentially means how we care for and dispose of our clothes.

- Between 75 and 80 percent of our clothing's impact comes from washing, drying, and ironing.

- The world now consumes about eighty billion new pieces of clothing every year. This is 400 percent more than the amount we consumed just two decades ago.

- As new clothing comes into our lives, we also discard it at a shocking pace—eleven million tons per year in the United States alone, which boils down to eighty-two pounds for the average American.

- Even though much of our clothing is made from "natural" fibers, it can take as long as forty years for them to decompose in landfills. And shoes can take up to a thousand years due to the use of an especially persistent synthetic material called ethylene vinyl.

However, we can change this! Ninety-five percent of clothing that ends up in landfills can be reused or repurposed in some way, which is beyond frustrating in retrospect, but it presents a real opportunity as we look forward to the responsible innovations that will shape and define fashion's future. Circularity is the new black. Even H&M has committed to being 100 percent circular and renewable by 2030. Check out their "Vision and Strategy" on their website. Here are some ways you too can take action:

- As garments wear over time, invest in having them repaired, resized, or updated to extend their life cycle.
- Check out and support RenewalWorkshop.com, where you can buy top brands such as Prana and Indigenous that have been refurbished to look like new, at lower prices than their current retail offerings.
- Host or attend a clothing swap. One person's trash is another's must-have-*IT* item.

- Avoid dry-clean only items altogether.
- Wash clothing only when soiled, and not automatically after every wear.
- Wash in cold water on the shortest cycle, or hand wash.
- Always run a full load of laundry.
- Hang laundry to dry instead of using the dryer.
- Use a concentrated, natural, nontoxic detergent, free of SLS (sodium lauryl sulfate), petroleum distillates, and synthetic fragrances.
- Donate old clothes, even the intimates you're inclined to discard. What's still wearable will be reworn and what's too tattered will have the best chance of being properly recycled or repurposed.

Purchase timeless, heirloom pieces that are made well. And don't throw textiles in the trash! Find somewhere to recycle them.

—Amber Valletta

Though style can be defined in a myriad of ways and can take on infinite incarnations, we can all agree that the beauty and value of a garment multiplies infinitely when we can be proud of where it comes from. Ethical fashion is a way to not only feel good about ourselves in the mirror, but also to positively affect the global fashion community and show a greater respect for our planet's precious resources. We all get dressed. Each one of us has a voice. And each of us can play a part in catalyzing the changes that are long overdue. On the other side of this destruction, there is an industry where diversity is celebrated, where transparency is a given, where people are valued well above profit, and where creativity doesn't come at the cost of the environment or human life. As my friend Harvey Russack of Green Shows agrees, "We must wear the change."

> Ethical fashion is a way to not only feel good about ourselves in the mirror, but also to positively affect the global fashion community and show a greater respect for our planet's precious resources.

The ECOrenaissance movement is all about living cohesively, developing a lifestyle that's supportive on both internal and external levels. Embracing organic farming methods for both food and fashion is an important component of this lifestyle. And while organic, ethically made clothing may seem like a big leap from the current state of the industry, it's been steadily gaining ground, and so many cutting-edge companies use organic fiber as a basic prerequisite for assurance of quality and consciousness. And, as it gains more and more support at the mainstream level, it will be nothing but win-win-win on every side. Any good designer knows that fashion is not purely utilitarian—it's a reflection of identity, both cultural and personal. It contains profound messages, and has a deep psychological impact on how people relate to themselves and interact with the world around them.

If we're carelessly consuming clothes made in ways that are inhumane and harmful to the environment, how does that affect our relationship with ourselves? How does it skew our priorities, desensitize us to the suffering of others? People grow and sew our products, and their lives are being affected. On a less immediate level, ours are too—our own choices are destroying us on both environmental and personal health levels. Moving toward conscious purchasing habits, cultivating and curating a wardrobe with a story you can be proud of, will make you glow from the inside out.

Imagine if, when it came to fashion, all our stories were positive. In my opinion, the green movement has historically put people off by embodying a preachy, fatalistic tone, leaving people feeling hopeless instead of activated. I have always believed that the way to ignite action is to inspire in a positive way. My film series with Amber Valletta and Tree Media, *Driving Fashion Forward*, pulled the curtain back on the industry, but with a positive lens.

We talked about the forward-thinking innovators who are doing amazing things within the industry, and told their stories as to why they're doing those things. The damaging effects of this industry are very real, but we have to think in terms of solutions, and cocreate a world where sustainability and beauty go hand in hand all the time. The Gandhi quote that kicked off this chapter expresses a powerful revelation.

At the rate we're going, we'll need two Earths by 2030, which is why our largest and most adored major corporations, such as C&A and Target, are jumping on the sustainability bandwagon. Target has nine main sustainability goals, and they're committed to the following in their responsible sourcing strategies:[16]

- Improving worker well-being; enhancing worker safety; eliminating forced labor.
- Achieving net positive manufacturing, including removing unwanted chemicals, optimizing water use, and driving clean energy.
- Deriving key raw materials from ethical and sustainable sources: sustainably managed forests and palm oil, responsibly grown and harvested cotton, and recycled polyester.

Now more than ever, it's important that we focus on original, relevant design that's engineered to be reused, recycled, or repurposed.

—Julie Guggemos

For Designers: Tips from Teslin Doud

Teslin is a social innovator and Parsons Award–winning Parsons School of Design graduate formerly from Eileen Fisher who helped drive their ecosystem through Remade in the USA, an incredible recycling and take-back program. She has these tips to share with current and future fashion designers:[17]

- Consider a product's next life as you design its first life.
- A little extra work now allows for efficiency later.
- How will the information about a product be available for its next designer?
- Design your process, not just your product.
- How will your product tell its story?

Call to action for ECOrenaissance readers: bring your clothing back to Eileen Fisher and learn about its continued life story. Eileen Fisher has committed to being a 100 percent sustainable company by 2020!

Solving today's major environmental threats demands a closer look not just at the ways products are made and from what materials, but at the entire supply chain ecosystem that produces them. We need to create the new.

—**Cyrill Gutsch**

Additional Resources for Designers, Makers, Brands, and Retailers

Brooklyn Fashion Design Accelerator (BFDA)
Common Objective
Copenhagen Fashion Summit
Ecospire
Fair Fashion Center at Glasgow Caledonian University
Fashion for Good
Sustainable Apparel Coalition
Textile Exchange

The DNA of ECOrenaissance Fashion: No Compromise in Style or Substance

- Ethical: no child labor; safe working conditions; fair trade/living wages for farmers and workers.
- Support conscious brands and curated ECOfashion websites; join sustainable fashion communities (refer to the resources list in this chapter and at the back of this book).
- Sustainable/organic fibers and materials.
- No toxic chemicals in dyeing and processing, such as formaldehyde and chlorine bleach, as well as heavy metals.
- Water/energy conservation (renewables) in production and home care (wash in cold water).
- Slow fashion: reduce, reuse, rent, recycle; waste management/zero waste; circular economy; vintage; buy less.
- Collaborate with others to drive innovation.
- Connect around fashion in a positive way: share, repurpose, and make your own.
- Look good, feel good, do good in the world.

Illuminartist Interviews: *Fashion*

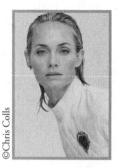

©Chris Colls

Amber Valletta, Supermodel
www.ambervalletta.com

Truly gorgeous from the inside out, Amber epitomizes a role model like no other. She walks the talk and talks the walk, so follow her on the runway and beyond. Be sure to watch our documentary series *Driving Fashion Forward with Amber Valletta*.

What is a personal ECOrenaissance tip you can share with readers?

Purchase timeless, heirloom pieces that are made well. And don't throw textiles in the trash! Find somewhere to recycle them.

Which of the pillars of the ECOrenaissance movement (collaboration, consciousness, community, creativity, connection) resonate most with you and why?

All of them! They're all interconnected and necessary to create meaningful change in fashion and beyond.

What is your vision for the future of fashion?

My wish for fashion's future is that sustainability is viewed as a norm—it's simply integral to every decision made along the supply chain, from the raw materials to the designers to the retailers to the consumers. Circular fashion is the direction in which we must all go.

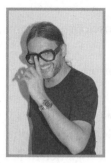

Cyrill Gutsch, Founder of Parley for the Oceans
www.parley.tv/#fortheoceans

An ocean crusader who has fused brilliant design into innovative action, Cyrill is paving the way for an end to plastic pollution. From Adidas to Stella McCartney, brands worldwide are joining this amazing man's vision at Parley for the Oceans.

What is a personal ECOrenaissance tip you can share with readers?

It's a myth that environmental responsibility demands sacrifice. You don't have to be a martyr or a purist to own your impact and drive positive change. Every breath you take is generated by the oceans. And every decision you make is an opportunity to start living in acknowledgment of that fact. Anyone can implement the Parley AIR Strategy—Avoid, Intercept, Redesign—by first avoiding single-use plastics such as bags and bottles. Items we use once and discard are made from a material that lasts forever, that ends up on beaches, in the bellies of sea life, in our own bloodstreams. If you have access to alternatives, use them. If you don't, demand them. Or better: create them.

How did you start your journey toward sustainability/social purpose?

I can pinpoint the turning point in my career to a conversation I had in June 2012, when I met Captain Paul Watson, founder of Sea Shepherd Conservation Society and cofounder of Greenpeace. He was being held in Germany at the time, under attack for defending defenseless sea life in the oceans. It was shocking. I thought, here's this altruist pirate being treated like a criminal for protecting the life that ensures our own survival. Through Paul, I learned that if we don't turn this around, if we're not the generation that fixes this, the legacy we leave behind will be a dead ocean. I couldn't accept that. It didn't just change my mind-set; it changed my life.

Prior to meeting Captain Paul, I focused my career on helping struggling brands and companies turn around. Once I learned what was happening in our oceans, I had to act. I took on a new project with the ultimate deadline, making the oceans my biggest and most important client yet. I founded Parley for the Oceans to create a space and network for members of the creative industries to have the same epiphany—and more importantly, to act on it.

Which of the pillars of the ECOrenaissance movement (collaboration, consciousness, community, creativity, connection) resonate most with you and why?

Creativity, collaboration, eco-innovation. That's the formula for solutions. We cannot solve massive, complex problems such as plastic pollution with the same dated thinking, flawed materials, and siloed decision-making that created them. If we allow sea life to go the way of the dinosaurs, our species will be close behind. We can fix this, but we need to harness our imaginations and invent our way out. And we need to work together to get there.

What is your vision for the future of fashion?

There will be no future of anything if we fail to make peace between the economic system of humankind and the ecosystem of nature. At Parley, we're negotiating the peace agreement through our strengths as humans: eco-innovation, creativity, collaboration. We have a strategy—Parley AIR—and a symbol. Together with Adidas, we developed a material from upcycled marine plastic waste that can replace virgin plastic: Parley Ocean Plastic. This is a proof of concept and an invitation, a call to action to set new standards and create the next step forward. It's also a huge business opportunity. It can be more lucrative to protect the oceans than it is to destroy them. This is the way forward.

The industry is already changing. It's not enough anymore to have a beautiful product or experience, or to simply check the boxes on a CSR report. Every item tells a story, and as people become increasingly educated and aware of the threats to our planet, they want to feel they're not just supporting what is right but participating in it. No brand exists in isolation. Solving today's major environmental threats demands a closer look not just at the ways products are made and from what materials, but at the entire supply chain ecosystem that produces them. We need to create the new. The decisions we make now will shape the planet for generations. In this evolving landscape, purpose is the new luxury.

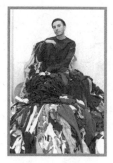

Daniel Silverstein, Fashion Designer
www.zerowastedaniel.com

Daniel is one of my favorite all-time designers. I've been proud to grace red (and green) carpets worldwide in our fabulous ECOfashion cocreations. Visit his website to learn more and support his mission for a zero-waste fashion world!

What is a personal ECOrenaissance tip you can share with readers?

I make the whole thing a game. Hunt for the least packaged items, check labels for the most local products, and see if you can find an alternative to single-use and disposable products. It's as simple as keeping a fork with you.

How did you start your journey toward sustainability/social purpose?

It was less of a how, and more of a how could I not? In school I was clued in to some of the pollution and waste in the world. There's no way I could start a business or even do things as simple as grocery shopping without taking these factors into account. I'm far from perfect in my quest for zero waste, but just trying to stay mindful and responsible has exponentially reduced my impact over the last five years.

What is your vision for the future of fashion?

I believe in reeducating consumers and the millennial workforce about labor. Let's get our hands dirty and rebuild the industry from the ground up.

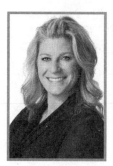

Julie Guggemos, SVP Product Design and Development for Target
www.target.com

Having collaborated with Target for more than a decade, I'm thrilled by Julie's leadership and the engagement and vision of the Target product design and development teams. This company has real power to influence and effect lasting change at a mass level. Go Julie!

How did you start the journey toward sustainability/social purpose and why?

Throughout my career, I have worked with and learned from design leaders at Target and around the world, and it has become apparent that a sustainable approach to design is the only option in today's world. Making good design choices to better the world is inspiring to my team and me. Twenty years from now, I want to look back and know we made a positive impact in our communities and on our planet.

Which of the pillars of the ECOrenaissance movement (collaboration, consciousness, community, creativity, connection) resonate most with you and why?

To me it's not about isolating any one of the ECOrenaissance elements, rather it's about combining them to bring about a more innovate approach. I love the idea of bringing the community together, along with designers, to collaborate and cocreate solutions to make the world a better place to live.

What is your vision for the future of fashion?

Runways are becoming real-time, vintage is cool, and the millennial consumer is choosing experiences and/or products with shared value sets over stuff. Now more than ever, it's important that we focus on original, relevant design that's engineered to be reused, recycled, or repurposed. It's our responsibility as a design team.

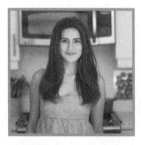

Lauren Singer, *Trash Is for Tossers* Blog; Founder of Simply Co.
www.trashisfortossers.com
www.thesimplyco.com

You must follow this zero-waste power woman on social media. Lauren is not only one of the most cool and conscious influencers I know, but her Package Free Shop (see packagefreeshop.com) is an amazingly innovative model for the future of retail.

What is a personal ECOrenaissance tip you can share with readers?

When it comes to lessening personal impact, I believe that any positive change is positive. I don't think there is a *one size fits all* place to start when it comes to sustainability, and so I suggest thinking about one alternative that helps to reduce a single-use item in your life, something easy, and then commit to it. For instance, do you use plastic forks with your takeout lunch? How about carrying a reusable fork every day. Do you get coffee in a single-use plastic cup? Try bringing along a reusable one. They might seem like small changes, but that's okay! Everything that we can do, no matter how small, to decrease the amount of waste we're producing is positive. Who knows—that one simple, little thing that becomes part of your routine could empower you to make more and more lifestyle choices to reduce your impact and you might even end up like me, making your own laundry detergent and then one day quitting your job to start your own company!

What is your vision for the future of fashion, business, and/or entertainment?

My goal in life is to help create positive environmental change. Every choice I make is guided by that sentiment. Whether it is empowering people to reduce their own personal impact, or starting a company to solve problems within the consumer product space, there is always work to be done. My vision is that we move away from plastics, landfills, fossil fuels, combustion engines, single-use items and packaging, preserved and packaged "food products," large-scale agriculture, and planned obsolescence and toward a future that resembles the world before we had these things, but with modern luxuries provided by sustainable technology and renewable energy. I have no doubt that through the ingenuity of some amazing thinkers and entrepreneurs, this will happen.

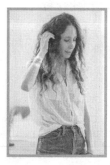

Mara Hoffman, Fashion Designer
www.marahoffman.com

A living example of marrying one's personal and professional values, Mara Hoffman has taken the fashion industry by storm with her design talent, vision, and passion for positive change. I know firsthand that in Mara's designs, looking good has never felt so good.

Which of the pillars of the ECOrenaissance movement (collaboration, consciousness, community, creativity, connection) resonate most with you and why?

I think all five are super important, but consciousness, creativity, and connection resonate the deepest.

Consciousness, because I don't think you can really make a lasting change without feeling it on a deep level and feeling it as a part of your consciousness. Without that feeling, it would be fleeting, wavering, something that's easy to turn on and off.

Creativity is about finding ways around obstacles, rethinking things, being creative within every moment of change. Change takes creativity and then connection to implement that change on a wider scale.

The connection is about reaching out to the community for resources and then connecting with our peers and people who are further down the road than we are within this process, and in turn, reaching our hand out to those who are less traveled down the road. I believe if you're sincerely in this, you're in it for everybody. You're not just in it to see yourself rise in the world of sustainability, which would go against the entire consciousness of the movement. If we want it, we want for every single one of us to be doing it. It's the only way it will work.

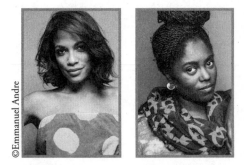

©Emmanuel Andre

Rosario Dawson (with Abrima Erwiah), Fashion Brand and Retailer/Actress
www.studiooneeightynine.com

Rosario has inspired us onscreen, and now she's working her magic as a change maker and advocate of the fashion revolution. Ask Rosario, "Who made your clothes?" and she'll proudly let you know at her incredible new store with her soul sister Abrima.

What is a personal ECOrenaissance tip you can share with readers?

It's about putting people and the planet first. It's simple gestures like asking yourself: Who made my clothes? Who participated in the making of my clothes? The farmers? Their children? The cleaning people? The transporters? The weavers? Every single person that participated in allowing you the opportunity to wear your clothes. What is your relationship to them? Do you honor them by honoring the clothes you're wearing? Do you think about their living conditions? Their feelings? Do you ever wonder what their names are? Ask yourself when you're consuming: Are you consuming your fair share? What happens to other people when we overconsume? Where does our waste go?

I just think it's really asking yourself simple questions and considering the lives of the people you may be affecting by the choices you make. We do not exist independently. We have one planet, we are one world, and we have to share it. I think if you consider the people and the planet when you make purchasing decisions or decide how much and what to consume, then that's already a huge feat. It's about making the invisible visible.

A simple gesture would be to buy quality products that are built to last instead of buying trendy items. And if you buy products that you expect to wear only a few times, participate in a clothing swap with your friends or in your community so that your excess clothing doesn't end up in landfills, in the water, etc.

Another simple gesture is asking yourself who made your clothes and asking the brands that you're consuming to answer that question. Shop at small businesses, shop for locally produced goods. Know and wear your impact.

How did you start your journey toward sustainability/social purpose?

We started our journey in Bukavu in the Democratic Republic of the Congo, at the opening of the City of Joy (COJ) in 2011. The COJ is a leadership center for women who have been the victim of rape and sexual violence. Opened by V-Day, Eve Ensler's organization is dedicated to stopping violence against women and rape. Rosario sits on the board of V-Day and invited me [Abrima Erwiah] to join the opening of the COJ. It was a very challenging trip that took us from New York to Philadelphia to London to Kenya to Burundi to Rwanda and finally to Bukavu. Despite how difficult our journey was to get to Bukavu (for reasons too long to explain here), when we arrived we met the most amazing women who had been through so much trauma but were still smiling and happy. These women built the city themselves. And not only that, they also made crafts, and they would sell their crafts and take the proceeds and invest in agriculture. They would farm products like cassava, for example, and use the agricultural products to feed their kids and the proceeds from the sale of their agricultural products to send their kids to school.

We saw this beautiful circle of sustainability happen. We saw that theirs was the existence of microeconomies in villages such as these and we just knew. We knew this was our purpose. Our purpose was to create a platform, a space to empower those who were already doing amazing work to develop and to help them build their businesses. We had the dream of Studio 189 years before, but it was this trip where we were called, and we knew it was our time to answer.

Which of the principles of the ECOrenaissance movement (collaboration, consciousness, community, creativity, connection) resonate most with you and why?

All the principles resonate but we will speak of collaboration for the purposes of replying to this question. There is a traditional West African *adinkra* symbol called *Boa me, boa na me mwoah*. It means "Help me and let me help you." It's a traditional symbol of collaboration and interdependency. We use it as a symbol representing how we work. We believe in the power of collaboration. We believe in the power of people working together, that no one person is better than another, and that if we work together and learn from each other and transfer skill sets, we can all rise together for a better world.

What is your vision for the future of fashion?

The future of fashion is global and local. It's about understanding local needs, supporting local demand, and creating goods locally where possible, allowing us to reduce the hidden cost of fashion's environmental, social, political, and economic impact.

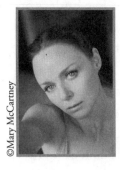

©Mary McCartney

Stella McCartney, Fashion Designer

www.stellamccartney.com

Stella is a world-leading designer and human who has tirelessly championed health, wellness, and a sustainable lifestyle at every turn. A Michelangelo of the ECOrenaissance, Stella has designed a new reality in the spirit of the greater good—an inspiration to all.

What is your vision for the future of fashion?

I'm in fashion and I don't use leather, fur, or PVC. This is unheard of. It's really become my point of difference. This is an industry based on selling leather, you go into stores and you're hit by handbags, not by ready-to-wear. I was always told that I'd never have an accessory business because people associate leather with luxury. But I'm approaching it in a different way. We're the only luxury house providing this kind of product and proving it's doable. It's the most game-changing thing we've done in the industry. This is what drives me, challenges me, and defines the modernity of my brand. The use of leather for fashion has a massive environmental impact. Massive. From unnecessary water consumption to high emissions of greenhouse gases and polluting chemicals.

So for me it's really about questioning the process. Fashion has to modernize. It has to challenge its history. More than fifty million animals a year are killed in the name of fashion, and that has to stop. It's not ethical, responsible, or sustainable. For me it's the most exciting challenge. I can design a dress that people dream of in three months' time. I can be modern and on trend in that sense, but actually beyond all that there's a different kind of modernity that's driving me, in partnership with great design. It's a really interesting layer that's added into the way that I work and a different way of doing things. It's about the bigger picture, about the future of our world, and how we can help impact that!

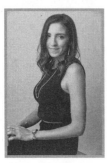

Stephanie Cordes, Cordes Foundation
www.cordesfoundation.com

Finding her calling and leveraging her passion for sustainable fashion through impact investments, Stephanie's leadership and vision as forces for change will help manifest a new chapter in ECOfashion.

What is a personal ECOrenaissance tip you can share with readers?

Accessorize. Rather than buying new outfits for every occasion I recommend investing in a sustainably produced capsule collection along with ethically made statement accessories. This gives you the ability to mix and match pieces in order to create entirely new looks while still achieving standout, sustainable, and effortlessly chic style.

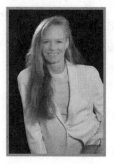

Suzy Cameron, Founder of Red Carpet Green Dress
www.redcarpetgreendress.org

Leader of the ECOwarrior fashionistas, Suzy's vision to turn the red carpet to green has been unparalleled. With her fellow plant-based creative genius husband, James Cameron, this couple is *the* quintessential ECOrenaissance king and queen. Invest in the next generation and support Suzy's amazing green school for K–12 at museschool.org.

What is a personal ECOrenaissance tip you can share with readers?

There's an elegant solution: eat at least one plant-based meal a day for the planet. Animal agriculture—that's the meat and dairy we eat—is the second leading cause of greenhouse gas emissions, which is more than all of transportation combined! It's also the leading driver of ocean dead zones, deforestation, and extinction. The more of a plant-based diet you eat, the lighter your "food print." In fact, if the United States ate 50 percent less meat, it would be equivalent to taking twenty-six million cars off the road. The bottom line: it's a win for the environment and a win for your health and well-being.

What is your vision for the future of fashion?

I'm working toward a world where everything we eat and wear is contributing to a thriving ecosystem, not damaging or extracting from our environment. I hope "fast fashion" will be just a bad dream, and that sustainably produced and socially conscious fashion is the norm, accessible to all.

7

Conscious Business
and Consumerism

> No problem can be solved from the same level
> of consciousness that created it.
> —ALBERT EINSTEIN

Every topic we've been exploring in this book so far ultimately comes down to changing business models and expanding our power as consumers. Everything we buy affects other people's lives. Our food doesn't grow in the supermarket, and our clothing isn't produced in department stores. We've been living with a counterintuitive system, and it's no longer working. But if we take the example of the multitude of emerging companies that foster radical change *while* achieving mainstream success, we can see that businesses have the power to do just as much good as, historically, they have done harm.

Every topic we've been exploring in this book so far ultimately comes down to changing business models and expanding our power as consumers.

One proponent for this stance is Andrew Winston, my dear friend and a globally recognized expert on how companies can navigate and profit from humanity's biggest challenges. Referencing his new book, *The Big Pivot*, he shared with me that megatrends are changing the world in profound ways and deeply challenging how we do business by offering:[1]

- Strategies for dealing with a changing (and increasingly expensive) climate that brings extreme weather and disrupts business operations around the world.
- Dramatically cheaper clean energy and technologies.
- Continuing pressure on and competition for natural resources (such as water).
- Methods to meet the higher expectations of the millennial generation for corporate responsibility and meaning and purpose at work.
- Fast-changing technologies—big data, artificial intelligence, and more—that enable radical transparency about every product, service, and company.

Andrew told me, "Society is expecting ever more from business on climate, inequality, resource issues, and much more. The companies and executives that understand these profound changes will profit and thrive. Managing in this more complex, demanding environment requires a shift in focus, strategies, and tactics that I call the Big Pivot. It's no longer enough to make a safe product and just maximize shareholder value this quarter. Successful companies focus instead on innovating to solve the world's challenges, and then using the powerful tools of capitalism and markets to do it most profitably. The true leaders are making three big pivots:

1. **The vision pivot:** Challenge the short-term focus that makes it hard to invest in the business for the long term; set goals tied to what science tells us the world needs (such as the hundred-plus multinationals that have committed to 100 percent renewable energy); and innovate in new ways by asking disruptive, heretical questions about the business (e.g., Nike and Adidas investing in new 'dry dyeing' technologies after asking, 'Why do we need water to dye clothes?').
2. **The valuation pivot:** Rethink how to incentivize employees with meaning and rewards for building sustainable enterprises; make better investment decisions by taking into account the broader return on sustainability (such as attracting and retaining top talent, enhancing customer loyalty, and building brand value); and put a value on the natural capital of business and society we rely on.
3. **The partner pivot:** Work in new ways with customers, competitors, and suppliers to innovate and manage the impacts of the business, and encourage the government by lobbying *for* rules that protect the climate and drive sustainability."[2]

In his own words, Andrew recognizes that "the world is heading toward a global population of nine or ten billion people, all wanting a higher quality of life, and all demanding more of companies. We face increasing resource stress and dangerous, expensive climate change, but business can lead the charge. We have most of the technological solutions we need—we just need leaders to make the pivot. It's time for business to step up and build a thriving world."

As a kid with business cards by age eleven, I have always had a deep passion for business, knowing that it can be harnessed as an extraordinary force for good—often even more powerful than government. As consumers, we can "vote" with our dollars for products that make us look and feel better from the inside out, all the while supporting social well-being and a thriving environment.

> As consumers, we can "vote" with our dollars for products that make us look and feel better from the inside out, all the while supporting social well-being and a thriving environment.

The paradigms are shifting. We're starving for authenticity and transparency, and corporations are responding. For decades, companies have been operating around a faster-cheaper-more mentality, thinking in terms of immediate gratification without regard to greater impacts. And until relatively recently it was entirely possible to do this. Before the Internet, there was no easy way to research a company's practices—we just had to trust what was being advertised to us. But with the ever-expanding accessibility of the Internet, now anyone can gain greater awareness into the nature of the products they're purchasing, and ask game-changing questions:

- Who made this?
- How was it made?
- Is it serving the environment or hurting it?
- How will consuming this product affect my health and well-being?

It's only getting easier and easier to find the answers. Thanks to this heightened awareness, the ECOrenaissance is witnessing an absolute boom in new, groundbreaking, conscious companies. And these businesses are flourishing because they're connecting with consumers at a core level, giving us what we actually desire, need, and crave, with no compromise necessary. In this chapter we'll talk about how to engage your buying power to support conscious businesses, how to find these companies, and how we can all participate in a thriving, sustainable economy by finding love and passion in our work.

I think if in every sector of industry we considered what's good for our children and future generations, as the indigenous peoples of the world did, the earth and its resources would be used more sustainably and responsibly.
—**Laura Turner Seydel**

Voting with Your Dollars

Everything we buy has an impact. Our day-to-day purchasing activity communicates directly to the economy and shapes how businesses serve and supply our demands. We can take an active part in shifting local and global industries in a positive direction. As consumers, it's time to step up and embrace our power.

- **Start small.** Is there a choice you can make that's better, more informed? If you're going to buy bottled water, is there a brand you can buy with a bio-degradable bottle? If you're going to use sunscreen, is there a brand available with fewer toxic chemical ingredients? If you're going to buy groceries, can you avoid plastic bags? What's the best you can do, in *your* particular situation, in *this* moment? Every moment is a rebirth. Every moment is a choice full of new possibilities.

- **Get informed.** Think of the products, industries, and issues you're interested in and the resources available to you. There are a lot of certifications that make buying smart and sustainable easy (on which we will go into more detail later in this chapter). There's also a wealth of information about the company or product in question—progressive companies will have detailed information on their websites, and third-party resources (such as the Think Dirty app for cosmetics) contain a wealth of information. If all else fails, google a company or product that you're curious about and start from there.

- **Think long-term.** A lot of people automatically reach for the cheaper option, without thinking about what they're actually spending their money on. Would you pay a little more if you knew that you were getting much more value—if the product was higher quality, longer lasting, and sustainably and ethically produced? In the long run, isn't it worth it?

- **It's not all-or-nothing.** Allow the information to sink in. Let yourself be where you are. I've spoken to many people who are apprehensive about engaging with conscious buying habits at all because they're afraid of feeling hypocritical if they don't do everything perfectly. Remember, this isn't a race to enlightenment, but a journey—the little things really do add up, and after a while it becomes intuitive.

As human beings, at our core we all want to do good. No one sets out to consume products that are harmful and destructive, of course—those products have simply seemed like the most available, affordable choices. In the past, most people didn't even really realize they *had* a choice to begin with. But this is all changing as society is waking up and discovering endless possibilities within business that allow for products that are not only sustainable and ethical but also affordable, creative, fun, and stylish. And now it's no longer about why *would* you support these companies; the question is, why *wouldn't* you?

We vote with our pocketbooks. So if you want a cleaner, safer, healthier planet one must put their hard-earned money where their mouth is.
—Rachelle Carson Begley

No Compromise: Value and Values

When I was starting out in ECOfashion, people automatically equated conscious consumerism with compromise, assuming that healthy food couldn't also taste good, fashion couldn't also be environmentally friendly, and successful companies couldn't also maintain ethical practices. Here's why that line of thinking is wrong:

- As I shared in the previous chapter, what I quickly learned was that *on an economic level, no-compromise business practices make much more sense*. As noted in the chapter on fashion, by going straight to the source, cutting out unnecessary middlemen and the price markups that accompany them, businesses can add sustainability and quality *while* cutting costs.

- Second, conscious business resonates with consumers. Little to no marketing is needed because the products speak for themselves. When my cofounder and I first opened Gulliver's Living & Learning Center, we would always tell our customers, "Don't believe anything we say, just try it." Consumers are craving *authenticity and purpose*, and when companies are able to deliver on those principles while also exceeding expectations in terms of quality, there is absolutely no substitute.

My peers in the industry all understand that these conscious companies are thriving because they're filling a fundamental human desire for meaning and purpose. When real passion is apparent in a brand, it's irresistible. Love creates strong business, which has the power to heal, uplift, and transform our world.

I envision a world where I don't have to ask *if* something is safe, healthy, just, sustainable, organic, right, good, recycled—it simply *is*.
—Erin Schrode

New Conscious Business Models

Historically, the prototypical corporate marketing strategies would spend millions researching consumer behavior, trying to get inside their heads and manipulate, figuring out how to sell consumers things they didn't really want or need.

For example, my kids and I giggle about how much time, energy, and company dollars many brands spend trying to reach millennials—a generation known for their lack of concern about big houses and high-paying jobs, who would prefer to spend their money on experiences rather than material things. Advertising executives are completely mystified. Think about the countless articles and think-tank pieces that have been written about how this is a generation that's impossible to get through to.

But younger generations are actually simplifying—it's the older generations, and their business systems, that are complicating things! I've observed that the best way to reach younger consumers is through transparency, simplicity, and purpose.

Here are some examples of major brands that are breaking the mold—with incredible success:

- **TOMS Shoes:** TOMS offers a business plan that highlights social responsibility alongside a cool, well-made product. The company donates one pair of shoes to a person in need for every pair of shoes sold, and since beginning in 2006 has expanded to apply this for-profit, One-for-One business model to provide eyewear, freshwater, and safe birth services to those in need. Naturally, the success of TOMS was instantaneous, because it didn't *need* to use carefully calculated marketing techniques to reach consumers. Both its social mission and the quality of its product shone through and spoke for themselves.

- **Starbucks:** Howard Schultz, executive chairman and former CEO of Starbucks, was equally influential in creating social awareness and redefining the limitations of ethical business when he committed to ensuring that Starbucks produced only Fair Trade coffee. Suddenly the coffee industry and Fair Trade became synonymous in the eyes of the consumer, forcing his competitors to take note and act accordingly. This took the industry by storm, and made the American food and beverage industry reconsider how ethics and values rooted in sustainability could transform business for the better.

- **Patagonia:** This outdoor clothing manufacturer set a standard in the business world by revealing their social and environmental impacts to the public in an effort to reduce the informational barriers between companies and consumers. This radical transparency is a bold move that has in every sense set the standard for other businesses. In 2007 Patagonia launched the Footprint Chronicles to bring transparency to their supply chain and tell the stories that other brands typically don't tell. The Footprint Chronicles maps out the textile mills, sewing factories, and farms all over the world that Patagonia engages, proudly showcasing the extended network of contributors that supply their products. They go further, linking the supply chain map to the products themselves through a highly responsive website that also features comprehensive videos on the various innovative technologies used in their fabric recycling program, garment repair services, and lifetime product guarantees.

Not coincidentally, TOMS, Starbucks, and Patagonia are household names. These wildly popular brands are just three of the many shattering the myth that financial success has to come at the expense of morals. And as it becomes more and more clear that people are innately drawn to brands that are honest, transparent, socially and environmentally minded and forward-thinking, even long-standing corporations are changing their approaches. These industry shifts show so clearly how much power we have as consumers. Conscious business isn't a small, niche market anymore; consumer demand has actually created a new paradigm.

Did You Know?

Good business is about serving others, not profiting at the expense of people and planet. In fact, serving others was the original goal of corporations. The Love Summit (founded by rock-star millennial Samantha Thomas, leading environmental advocate and champion and dear friend John Perkins—author of the *New York Times* bestseller *Confessions of an Economic Hitman*—and Dan Wieden of Wieden+Kennedy, who created the Nike "Just do it" campaign) provides an excellent summary of the changing corporate mind-set over the years:

> Corporations in the United States were originally formed for the purpose of enabling activities that would improve societal standards of living. This included providing public services, developing infrastructure, creating jobs, and cultivating lasting business-consumer relationships.
>
> But in the 1970s, economist Milton Friedman came up with a new economic agenda, stating that the sole goal of business was to maximize corporate profits regardless of social and environmental costs. Since adopting this mind-set, we have created a world where less than 5 percent of people in the United States consume almost 30 percent of the planet's resources, while half of the world is on the verge of starving, or actually dying of starvation. This is not a model; it cannot be replicated by China, Russia, or any other country, no matter how hard they try.
>
> Milton Friedman's economic agenda has failed us. While it may appear in numbers that we have succeeded in increasing corporate profits, profit is only lasting when it has a reciprocal relationship with its environment. Evidence such as climate change, a diminishing middle class, and worldwide poverty—all largely produced by poor business practices—have created a questionable future for generations to come. Because people and the planet cannot sustain these practices, businesses that perform such activities can neither thrive nor sustain themselves in the long term.[3]

ECOfy: Doing Conscious Business

> The connection economy thrives on abundance. Connections create more connections. Trust creates more trust. Ideas create more ideas.
> —Seth Godin

Conscious businesses enhance people, planet, profit, passion, and purpose holistically for the long term. They add brand value by fusing price, performance, and purpose for today's conscientious consumer.

These businesses also can (and should) experience:

- Inspiring innovation
- Strong business growth
- Internal passion and respect
- Employee loyalty and integrity
- Drawing good talent
- Attracting capital
- Increased efficiency
- Supply chain productivity
- Improved brand image
- A sense of global community
- Positive stakeholder relations
- Saving money
- Competitive differentiation

How and Why?

- There is a shared vision of the common good.
- The stewardship of a company's bottom line has been redefined and improved.
- The company engages and benefits new generations.
- Stakeholders have aligned core values and positive connected interests.
- Employees are incentivized and motivated to cocreate and collaborate.
- Passion and purpose are the fuel that propel the company forward.
- Conscious leadership can enhance a company's foundation and long-term success.

> Through collaboration with corporate, public, and governmental sectors, we can create accountability and sustainability measures that will benefit human, animal, and planetary health.
>
> —**Susan Rockefeller**

Certified-Conscious Business

How can we find these companies? Certifications are really useful for helping us navigate which companies are actually making the commitment to serve people, planet, and purpose. Look for CSR, B Corp, Cradle to Cradle, Fair Trade, and Certified Organic. You've probably heard of at least a few of these, while some may still be unfamiliar. Let's go into more detail about what is required to qualify for each certification.

Corporate Social Responsibility (CSR)

CSR is defined as the voluntary activities undertaken by a company to operate in an economic, social, and environmentally sustainable manner. While the old-school model of corporate success was based on the bottom line, today a different way of thinking about business is developing, where what matters is not just profit but also a company's voice and sense of purpose and service to the community. And CSR is not just about fulfilling a quota—a company can't just use LED lightbulbs and then suddenly call themselves eco-friendly, because we can all see right through that!

When companies implement responsible practices both locally and internationally, everyone benefits. When companies operate in an economically, socially, and environmentally responsible manner, with transparency as a core value, their success only magnifies. Mitigation of social and environmental harm are becoming increasingly critical for business success abroad. As firms take advantage of global opportunities, there is an understanding that incorporation of responsible business practices into investments and operations abroad not only benefits the local economies and communities, but makes good business sense as well.

Mainstream Companies Embodying CSR
Apple
Dell
Disney
Google
Microsoft/LinkedIn
Tesla
Toyota/Lexus
Virgin

B Corp, Because There's No Planet B

The ultimate vision for the ECOrenaissance is for companies to aim to be the best in the world by being the best *for* the world. Others share this dream, and have begun to turn the dream into a community. This community is called B Corp, strengthened by a shared commitment to the pillars of the ECOrenaissance and bound by a declaration of *INTERdependence*.

In their own words, "B Corp is to business what Fair Trade certification is to coffee or USDA Organic certification is to milk." B Corp has come so far since their inception just a decade ago, having certified more than 2,500 companies from sixty-five countries and over 150 industries; all these companies are committed to people and planet just as much as profit, working together toward one unifying goal: to redefine success in business.

And the companies that boast the B Corp certification are not just next-generation start-ups—many major companies, such as Patagonia, have also joined the community that's redefining what a successful business can look like. This is the ultimate ECOrenaissance business model, using creativity, innovation, and the powerful influence of business to solve social and environmental problems. B Corp is leading a global movement of people using business as a force for good, encouraging others to "B the change" (bcorporation.net).

Some Mainstream B Corp Companies
Dansko
Eileen Fisher
Numi Tea

Patagonia
Seventh Generation

Cradle to Cradle

The earth's resources are not unlimited. But in spite of this, the historical business model has been a linear one, where we just keep taking and taking until it becomes physically impossible to take any more. This is the place we now find ourselves—without any thought to the ramifications, we have been poisoning our own air and water, and now we look around and are alarmed by the proliferation of natural disasters and public health epidemics. The whole system is broken, and as a result, we're finally rethinking the business model in its entirety.

Cradle to Cradle is about shifting from a linear to a circular mind-set, where we give back everything we have taken from the earth. This new paradigm is inherently sustainable because it's regenerative. It's a holistic, forward-thinking, zero-waste model that's built on the idea that we can rebuild and strengthen—we just need to close the loop, to give back and replenish what we have depleted from the earth.

I'm on the board of advisors for Cradle to Cradle's textile vertical initiative, Fashion Positive. As we've discussed, fashion's negative impact has been massive, so it's critical to drive change in the industry through Cradle to Cradle regenerative concepts. True to this idea, Fashion Positive measures material health, material reuse, water stewardship, renewable energy, and social justice (www.fashionpositive.org).

Examples of Mainstream Companies Embodying Cradle to Cradle
AVEDA
C&A (European retailer)
Interface (carpets)
Method (cleaning products)
Steel Case (furniture)

Founding MetaWear

In 2013, I founded MetaWear, the first sustainable, GOTS- (Global Organic Textile Standard) and Cradle to Cradle–certified fashion manufacturing company in North America. Using renewable energy at our factory in Virginia, we produce custom, certified-organic apparel and accessories. This is the factory of the future, truly fashion forward. MetaWear has embraced full transparency and a "true cost" mentality:

- Supporting organic and regenerative agriculture
- Producing made-in-the-United-States apparel from Texas-grown organic cotton
- Operating with a vertically integrated supply chain (our garments can be cut, sewn, dyed, and printed under one roof)
- Employing a turnkey plug-and-play manufacturing platform to "make sustainability easy" for our brand and retail customers

I share my business story to point out that once people get the hang of a new model, it's actually much easier and more straightforward than the conventional practices we're used to. We have unlocked the DNA code that can help transform the world (www.metawearorganic.com).

Fair Trade

The Fair Trade initiative was created to form a new method for trade. This method prioritizes equality and sustainability within the marketplace, seeking to empower and enrich the lives of farmers and workers worldwide. Starbucks is an example of a major corporation that has, from the get-go, espoused Fair Trade standards of social accountability, environmental responsibility, economic transparency, and high product quality. This business model is win-win-win, benefiting everyone from the farmers to the consumers. Now, in large part thanks to Starbucks' commitment to this model, Fair Trade is a deeply embedded term when people think about coffee.

But Fair Trade extends past the food and beverage industry—in fact, I helped write the very first Fair Trade textile certification with Fair Trade USA. In my many travels to India to work with cotton farmers, I have witnessed firsthand the direct benefits of certifications such as Fair Trade. At home in the United States, where consumer goods are overwhelmingly plentiful and many of us are completely removed from their production, it might be easy to think of a certification such as Fair Trade as just a peripheral benefit. But this certification is changing lives every day, fusing human values into global business (Fairtradeusa.com; Fairtrade.net; Fairtradefederation.org).

Top Mainstream Fair Trade Companies
> Ben & Jerry's
> Honest Tea
> Lush (makeup, personal care)
> Prana (apparel)
> Starbucks
> Ten Thousand Villages (retail)

Certified Organic

Certified Organic is a stringent certification process for producers of food and other ag-ricultural goods, including textiles. Certified Organic represents the ultimate good busi-ness model, benefiting people and planet while simultaneously increasing profit. When we support and demand this standard, we help ensure the safety of farmers and the health of their land, soil, and ecosystems, and we fortify our own vitality by prioritizing the consumption of food and fiber that are free of GMOs, pesticides, herbicides, and toxic chemicals. As we discussed in chapter 3, the conventional farming use of glyphosate in herbicides is now directly tied to the exponential rise in cancer and autism. Nonorganic agriculture is drastically weakening our planet and our immune systems—and given their increasing accessibility and affordability, Certified Organic products have now gone mainstream.

This is a truly thrilling time for organics, and enormous strides are being made at an actionable level. In the United States, a system known as the commodity checkoff col-lects capital to fund research and marketing for agricultural products. Prior to 2018, this program was promoting products in an overarching, generalized way with no distinction between organic and nonorganic agriculture. This meant that funds collected from or-ganic agricultural commodities would go toward the general agricultural marketing pool, partially subsidizing widespread ad campaigns for conventional products. But in 2016, the Certified Organic industry proposed the creation of a separate, distinctive checkoff program. If this proposal goes through (which will hopefully be the case by the time this book is published, or soon thereafter), the Certified Organic industry will generate thirty to forty million dollars per year for marketing and research. Already, the Certified Organic industry is exploding in popularity and ubiquity, but this revolution in policy will exponentially expand its reach.

This standard is win-win-win, and people are paying attention. In stark contrast to the state of the industry and level of interest just a few years ago, every room I walk into to talk about organics is packed. People recognize the changing ecosystem and financial paradigms and are searching for solutions. The Certified Organic business model is built on value-added agriculture and products, with authenticity and transparency at its core—along with soil, human, and planetary health—and slowly but surely, everyone is starting to speak that language. At double-digit industry growth rates for more than twenty consecutive years, with more demand than supply at the consumer level, and with poverty rates decreasing and household incomes increasing around organic agricultural pockets in rural America, Certified Organic is not only bipartisan, it's also *good* business (ota.com).

Some Great Mainstream Organic Companies
Amy's Kitchen
Annie's
Clif Bar
Dr. Bronner's
Earthbound Farms
Nature's Path
Stonyfield Farms

My vision for the future of business is one where silos and divisions no longer exist. Leadership is a shared responsibility and success is based on impacts, not just returns.

—**Gigi Chang**

The Love Economy

Work is love made visible.
—KAHLIL GIBRAN

The change is happening. As an entrepreneur, I have been living it for the past few decades, but I have also witnessed it happening on a larger scale. For example, I was on the original advisory board of the Sustainable Brands International conference, founded by KoAnn Vikoren Skrzyniarz. I have continued to attend over the past decade plus, and have observed the absolute explosion of interest in recent years. At first, companies would just send their sustainability marketing people—it felt like an empty, obligatory gesture, and the conference ended up more like a support group, with everyone venting about how little progress was being made. Frustration was the predominant energy. But now this conference is consistently sold out, buzzing with thousands of people. Everyone can feel the excitement in the air, and companies are no longer just going through the motions, but are so proud to be part of this flourishing collective movement.

There's a key ingredient here: people who work within the new, conscious model tend to love what they do. They tend to be excited, passionate, and proud. I love working in conscious business for that reason—not a day goes by that I'm not learning something new, powerful, exciting, and inspiring. As an ECOpreneur, I often feel like a little kid in a candy store—doing what I love, making a living, and changing the world. YES.

Every one of us can take part in the Love Economy. A general rule of thumb: people have greater success when they're doing what they love, because their work becomes part of them. It's simply intuitive. When we follow our hearts, we're connecting with our livelihoods. Work becomes a choice instead of a chore, something we look forward to, and consequently we excel at our work. Love is the secret ingredient to true success. When we embrace this mentality, merging our disparate sets of values and fusing love into everything we do, our professional lives begin to come together so seamlessly and authentically. When we fall in love with ourselves and with our work, we attract this same positivity in every area of our lives.

The Love Summit

As mentioned earlier in this chapter, in 2013, the groundbreaking business conference the Love Summit was founded for exactly this reason. Through his time working in corporate America, John Perkins witnessed firsthand the destruction and devastation brought about by an economic system that prizes maximum profits above all else and at the expense of social and environmental well-being. So he created the Love Summit to bring people together from various sectors of conscious business to demonstrate its transformative potential.

The goal of the summit "is to bring to light why loving is good business—how acting from a place of compassion will not only benefit society and the environment, but also our businesses and other institutions. Love can be the motivation behind business planning and work relationships, instead of fear and scarcity, the current underpinnings of a suffering economy and environment. The Love Summit demonstrates how we can:

- Use individual and collective action to transform our economic system into one that's based on a life economy.
- Create purpose-driven, heart-centered business models that mobilize the movement of sustainability globally and universally.
- Inspire a global culture of love in business and throughout the world."[4]

The global awakening that is the ECOrenaissance starts at the individual level, with people who have come alive and are living their truth every day. It's so important to engage with work that lines up with our values and speaks to our souls. If we work from the inside out, searching within ourselves to find what excites and activates us, people will pay attention. We're drawn in by an instinctual desire to live our fullest lives, and we can't help but be intrigued and enticed by people who have embraced their true selves and live with purpose.

> The global awakening that is the ECOrenaissance starts at the individual level, with people who have come alive and are living their truth every day.

It's for this reason that, whenever I interview anyone for my companies, I seek out passionate people who love what they do. In every interview, I ask candidates, "What is your dream job?" It's important for me to know what really excites them, and I have found that the people who are the most successful are those who are passionate about what they do. *Love is the DNA of the ECOrenaissance.* When we fuse love into everything we do, we're living in the flow.

Try This: Do You Love Your Job?

- Howard Thurman said, "Don't ask what the world needs. Ask what makes you come alive, and go do it. Because what the world needs is people who have come alive."[5] *What makes you come alive?*

- What do the outward actions of your leadership demonstrate to the world? Compassionate leaders are caring, thoughtful, and aware of how their business models treat their employees.

- If you could write your own job description, what would it be? If an answer doesn't immediately surface, do some digging. Set aside considerations of profit for a moment, and question what excites you daily.

- Do your job and daily responsibilities have a sense of compassion and care for others? Think about how you treat your colleagues and customers to determine if you create a compassionate workplace.

- Ask yourself these questions, then write and reflect on your answers:

  What do I like to read or watch?
  What blogs do I follow?
  What do I talk to friends and loved ones about?
  What topics do I gravitate toward?

  These are the kinds of simple self-explorations that can help all of us move toward a place of joy and passion in our work. And then don't just talk about it. Do it. Be it. Embrace it; activate that part of you, even if it's just in baby steps. But don't lie dormant, or the battery will die. You've got to rev up your engine if you want to drive.

Coming Together

My husband, Eric, and I had the honor of speaking at the 2016 Love Summit, high-lighting the power of love, collaboration, and cocreation when it comes to business. Eric and I are especially connected to this concept, as it has shown up in our life together time and time again. As two entrepreneurs in the conscious products industry who were consistently drawn together by what can only be explained as a force larger than our-selves, we found that, as a team, we're unstoppable. As individuals we're both ambitious, purpose-driven, optimistic, and intense, and prior to our relationship, we were both already heading successful businesses. But once we fused our abilities and ideas, harness-ing the power of togetherness, our creative capacity absolutely skyrocketed.

When Eric and I came together, we were both riding the roller-coaster low that some-times comes with entrepreneurship, having both recently exited our own companies. So when we started to collaborate, we were both in blind-faith mode. But what we discov-ered was that, by being completely aligned with each other and embarking on a journey into a new future with no fear, we formed the basis for a powerful energetic cocreation. From the get-go, I helped him build his burgeoning company I AM, which eventually collaborated with Under the Canopy once I returned to the helm. I also introduced Eric to the founder of Runa, which became one of his passion projects when he started his own consulting company.

Eric and I started to realize that our worlds were colliding on so many levels. In 2016, the work I had been putting all my energy toward for twenty-five years began to take off all at once, and I was in a state of constant, exhilarating movement. He and I started brainstorming, as we wanted to bring all our incredible shared energy together to create one lifestyle consulting collective, a one-stop shop for driving conscious business forward. Our principles would be built on people, planet, prosperity, passion, and purpose, and our categories would encompass every key category of the ECOrenaissance that has been discussed in this book.

From this mutual intention, BeyondBrands was born. We curated a supertribe of con-scious business leaders, a collective of people who base their livelihoods on going beyond the surface. Many of these people are our friends from the natural products industry who have weathered the decades-long storm of the conscious products industry and are now thriving as mainstream awareness grows exponentially. BeyondBrands is now a premier conscious consulting firm, and our clients range from start-ups wanting to avoid the learning curve by seeking out experts to billion-dollar companies interested in infusing awareness into their practices.

A majority women-owned business, we have experts all across the board—in total, we have twenty partners and more than seventy members of our collective advisory practice—and for each project, we curate an individual team. Many of our experts were individual consultants before joining BeyondBrands, and now are contributing to the collaborative leveraging of expertise, so that we all win together. We're connecting the dots across so many modalities of business, proving time and time again that the whole is greater than the sum of its parts.

Recently, we joined forces with a mission-driven private equity fund, New Crop Capital, which had conceptualized a disruptive plant-based seafood company but needed assistance in the execution. They had the finances and we had a shared big idea—in the plant-based food industry, there was a white space for delicious products that look and taste like seafood and provide similar benefits without any ramifications to sea life, the oceans, or human health. BeyondBrands supplied the creative brainpower, including two top chefs who had been executive chefs and educators at Whole Foods for many years and helped formulate groundbreaking plant-based products such as Daiya Cheese.

These powerhouse brothers—Chad and Derek Sarno—put their heads together to study the inner workings of every nutrient found in seafood and applied it to our plant-based products—using, for example, omega oils from algae instead of fish. We have created unbelievably delicious fish-free tuna, crab-free cakes, and versions of other tasty seafood products, all derived from gluten-free, GMO-free ingredients. Good Catch will be a game-changing and revolutionary brand; this is the beauty of collaboration, and the inevitable outcome of working with talented, mission-driven, passionate people who are motivated by their love for what they do and a commitment to the extraordinary power of business.

A Bright Future

The shift toward conscious, purposeful, love-fueled business is positively transformative for all of us. Conscious business is inclusive, so no one benefits at the *expense* of

> Applying sustainable practices in business is the best choice both for the planet and for the products being made.

others. Embracing consciousness, love, and unity can only result in a win-win, with no sacrifices necessary.

Applying sustainable practices in business is the best choice both for the planet and for the products being made. There is not a single downside to striving toward consciousness both as consumers and as creators—there are only positives all around. And this is the direction in which business is headed. It's the way of the future. In fact, the Natural Marketing Institute calculated that the conscious products industry was valued at $198 million in 2005, and projected that this number will have risen to exceed $1.5 trillion by 2020. But this

ECOfy: Be a Conscientious Consumer

Consumers hold a great deal of responsibility and power. We can vote with our hard-earned dollars to support the companies that are laying the foundation for our future. Conscientious consumerism is now more important than ever. We're on the fringe of mitigating the damage done and recapturing the vital relationship with our ecology. There are endless examples throughout this book of people who saw the light of the ECOrenaissance and changed their practices and behaviors. They took small yet powerful steps and built on them day after day, week after week, year after year. They became habitual, almost ritualistic, to the point where it's just how they live. Some ways in which conscientious consumers can engage their buying power include:

Foods/beverages
Household: cleaning products/laundry detergents/paper goods, bed and bath
    linens, mattresses, carpets, furniture, etc.
Pet products
Personal care products/cosmetics
Transportation: planes/trains/automobiles/bikes
Clothing/apparel
Electronics; appliances
Travel (vacations, hotels, etc.)

doesn't come as a surprise—when we're awake, aware, and informed, why would we choose anything else?

Today's consumers have so many choices that are enlightened and aligned. The seeds of consciousness have been planted and are beginning to bloom. If we keep watering and cultivating them, we will all be a part of a bountiful, beautiful harvest.

Be mindful, particularly when it comes to what you purchase. Do your research and pursue products whose impact, from production to give-back, aligns with your values and your personal style.
—**Lauren Bush**

The DNA of ECOrenaissance Conscious Business: No Compromise in Values

- Do well by doing good—the five p's: people, planet, passion, purpose, and prosperity.
- Stakeholder engagement includes sharing core values.
- Respect is a two-way street (employees, vendors/suppliers, customers, investors, etc.).
- Talk *with*, not *at*: creating ethical, engaging experiences.
- *Good* business means ecology plus economy.
- We're stronger together than we are apart.
- Redefining value must include true costs.
- Authentic and transparent practices and engagement are paramount.
- Win-win partnerships exist internally and externally—practicing "coopertition."
- Social innovation; ECOpreneurship.
- Measuring ESG (Environmental, Social, and Governance); impact investing.
- Solution-driven; mindful leadership; positive culture.

Illuminartist Interviews: *Conscious Business and Consumerism*

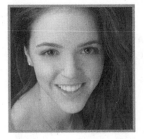

Erin Schrode, Founder of Turning Green
www.erinschrode.com
www.turninggreen.org

The youngest woman to ever run for the US Congress, Erin is a millennial superstar and game-changing ambassador for the planet and social justice. Follow her on social media!

What is a personal ECOrenaissance tip you can share with readers?

Why choose between beauty and health when you can have it all? Opt for safer and healthier cosmetics and personal care products, beginning with the universal essentials of soap, shampoo, deodorant, and toothpaste. Turning Green initially began as Teens for Safe Cosmetics, because of the link between the ingredients in daily-use products and cancer, birth defects, and reproductive harm. Learn to read labels: avoid chemicals listed on our Dirty Thirty; choose brands vetted for safety, sustainability, and efficacy.

What is your vision for the future of food, fashion, and lifestyle?

I envision a world where I don't have to ask *if* something is safe, healthy, just, sustainable, organic, right, good, recycled—it simply *is*. I envision a world where people think seven generations down the line, where education is prioritized, where transparency and authenticity are norms, where people and planet are valued alongside profit, where collaboration is paramount, where societies live in line with the natural bounty our planet provides.

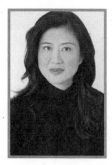

Gigi Chang, Founder of Plum Organics/Business Mentor
www.accelfoods.com

ECOpreneur and visionary, Gigi is now giving back to the next generation of innovators through her revolutionary food accelerator, go Gigi!

What is a personal ECOrenaissance tip you can share with readers?

Family dinner is an important part of our day. It's an opportunity to reconnect and share for all of us. To help set the right tone, I like to set the table and make sure the food is presented in a beautiful way. This includes cloth napkins, which are colorful and fun. It's a way to bring positivity to the end of a day and is more sustainable than paper napkins, which are used once and disposed of.

What is your vision for the future of business?

My vision for the future of business is one where silos and divisions no longer exist. People are hired based on their ability to learn and grow, not just experience or functional knowledge. Leadership is a shared responsibility and success is based on impacts, not just returns.

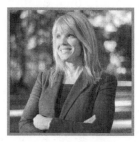

Laura Turner Seydel, Founder of Captain Planet Foundation
www.lauraseydel.com

In Laura's tireless and deeply dedicated work as a champion for the environment and our children's futures, she crosses multiple generations—inspired by her leading planetary advocate father, Ted Turner—and is passing the torch to the world at large.

What is a personal ECOrenaissance tip you can share with readers?

Aside from the oil industry, fashion retailers are among the top polluters in the world. Fortunately, there are committed, leading designers and companies providing more sustainable choices without sacrificing quality. We must support these businesses with our dollars. That is the most important thing we can do.

Which of the pillars of the ECOrenaissance movement (collaboration, consciousness, community, creativity, connection) resonate most with you and why?

Building awareness is absolutely critical in order to create the next cadre of environmental stewards. Obviously we can all participate in the simple things that demonstrate our commitment to protecting and restoring our communal life support system. For twenty-five years Captain Planet Foundation has filled an important niche and utilized all the ECOrenaissance principles to create the next generation of game changers and stewards of the environment. Our work is based on utilizing kids' natural creativity with place-based learning curricula to solve real-world problems. Collaboration with schools, administrators, educators, funders, parents, students, and nonprofits is key to the success of our programs, like Project Learning Garden and Project Hero.

What is your vision for the future of fashion, business, and/or entertainment?

I refer back to an old Native American proverb as the guiding light for my life and work: "We do not inherit the earth from our ancestors, we borrow it from our children." I think if in every sector of industry we considered what's good for our children and future generations, as the indigenous peoples of the world did, the earth and its resources would be used more sustainably and responsibly. If we considered their education, their quality of life, and their health first, we would change our practices. We would stop investing trillions of dollars in the art of war and invest in our children. We would stop polluting our water, and we'd stop treating our thin atmosphere as if it were an open sewer, dumping toxic, warming gases from the burning of fossil fuels. We would use the best sustainable practices in the growing of our food, instead of using chemical-intensive processes that kill living soil and expose families and communities to carcinogens.

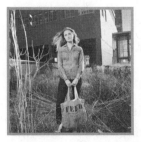

Lauren Bush, FEED Projects

www.feedprojects.com

Providing more than a hundred million meals to hungry children worldwide, Lauren epitomizes the humanity that connects us all. Her incredible efforts are the embodiment of the ECOrenaissance. Buy a super cool FEED bag, and FEED those in need. Win-win. Rock on, soul sister!

What is a personal ECOrenaissance tip you can share with readers?

Be mindful, particularly when it comes to what you purchase. Do your research and pursue products whose impact, from production to give-back, aligns with your values and your personal style. These products are out there. As consumers, we need to continue to demand products that make the world a better place. Harness your purchasing power.

What is your vision for the future of fashion and/or business?

I envision a future where fashion and businesses alike are much more socially, environmentally, and politically conscious and active. We're already seeing this happen, and I don't think it's going to slow down. Behind the fashion label and the business is a person, or a group of people, who have real interests and opinions and want to see a brighter tomorrow. They also know that today's consumer is pushing for products and purchasing options that are clean, ethical, and make a real difference. People desire more than just a bag or a scarf or a coffee, they want to know what that bag stands for, where it was made, what it was made from, and how it helped the world.

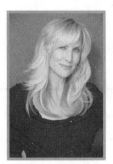

Rachelle Carson Begley, Actress/*Living with Ed Begley*

www.rachellecarson-begley.com

What's it like "Living with Ed"? The woman "behind" the man, Rachelle is the ultimate forward thinker, ecotrouper, actress, and advocate for the planet. Stylish and smart, she radiates true beauty on every level.

What is a personal ECOrenaissance tip you can share with readers?

We vote with our pocketbooks. So if you want a cleaner, safer, healthier planet one must put their hard-earned money where their mouth is. Now more than ever there are clean, safe, beneficial products on the market, from personal care products to clothing to home furnishings. I will say that just because something says it's sustainable doesn't always mean it is, so do a little research, and if that isn't your thing, refer to sites like Environmental Working Group or talk to friends you trust. Pretty much anything can be accessed on the Internet.

My husband, Ed Begley, and I just built a LEED Platinum Home in Studio City, California, and we're launching a site called BegleyLiving.com because we want to offer the knowledge and experience we acquired building our sustainable dream home. You actually *can* have it all. I have a beautiful home that's all solar and the latest sustainable technologies and beautifully designed. One really does not have to sacrifice style anymore for function. So I guess the best advice I can give is get educated on what sustainability really means and then do your best to have your lifestyle reflect your values. It's too important not to.

What is your vision for the future of fashion and lifestyle?

My vision for the future of fashion and lifestyle is a world where we don't have to choose between good and evil: goods are made sustainably by people who are paid a living wage and there doesn't have to be compromise. That people and the planet are held in the highest regard and that dictates our style, lifestyle, and creativity. Dreams become reality.

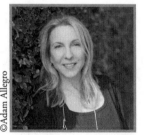

©Adam Allegro

Susan Rockefeller, Founder of Protect What Is Precious/ *Musings* Magazine

www.protectwhatisprecious.com

www.musingsmag.com

Entrepreneur, conservationist, and filmmaker, Susan is an inspirational changemaker actively dedicated to living an ECOrenaissance lifestyle. Sign up to receive her amazing publication at musingsmag.com!

What is a personal ECOrenaissance tip you can share with readers?

Like Michael Pollan says, "We all have the power to make a difference by voting with our forks three times a day." We should all educate ourselves on what we're eating and try to eat locally grown food as much as possible. Plant-based diets have much lower carbon footprints than those of meat, so even starting with a "meatless Monday" can be a significant contribution. The same line of thought applies to fashion. Know where your clothes are coming from and make conscious choices. Buy well-made, timeless pieces that you love and will wear often.

Which of the pillars of the ECOrenaissance movement (collaboration, consciousness, community, creativity, connection) resonate most with you and why?

All the principles resonate with me equally. I believe that they all need to work together in order to create a more sustainable, common future. I believe that a consciousness change through widespread education is key. Additionally, through collaboration with corporate, public, and governmental sectors we can create accountability and sustainability measures that will benefit human, animal, and planetary health.

What is your vision for the future of food and fashion?

My personal vision is that there will be an emergence of local hubs for innovation in food and fashion. People will have the opportunity to support and buy from local producers and brands. With more businesses participating in the circular economy and fulfillment of the sustainable development goals, global transnationals will play a part in producing goods and services (e,g., electronics, iPhones, food, etc.) that are more sustainably made and distributed.

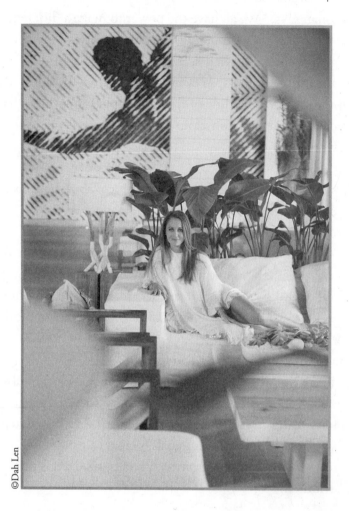

©Dah Len

This is one of the most stunning lobbies you'll ever see. Channeling my inner goddess at the eco-fabulous 1 Hotel South Beach—from the exquisite "Plant the Future" art and gorgeous reclaimed wood furniture to the eco-chic spa and über-cool organic juice bar—I feel like I'm in a no-compromise heaven on earth.

Conclusion

We but mirror the world. All the tendencies present in the outer world are to be found in the world of our body. If we could change ourselves, the tendencies in the world would also change. As a man changes his own nature, so does the attitude of the world change toward him. This is the divine mystery supreme. A wonderful thing it is and the source of our happiness. We need not wait to see what others do.

—MAHATMA GANDHI

Through the six ECOrenaissance modalities—art, food, wellness, beauty, fashion, business—and beyond, we're collectively experiencing a total rebirth. In the midst of so much darkness, a light has been ignited and is only shining brighter and brighter every day. The positive vibrations that originate within will circulate and radiate outward, creating a ripple effect that can impart joy and hope and change beyond what we ever imagined was possible.

As we unify our energy, creativity, and actions, we cocreate a new existence. Never doubt that this is possible—the fundamental nature of human beings is to innovate. With the exception of nature, we built everything we see around us, and we have the power and ability to devise a new reality that coexists effortlessly with our environment. But with creative capacity comes the propensity to destroy and harm, which is the path that humankind has often strayed down. If we stay on this path, if we live with blinders on, we *will* destroy everything around us—including ourselves.

There is no separation, and we exist as part of a massive concentric circle, where everything is self-contained. We all live under the canopy together. We all breathe the same air. And right now, people can't breathe because the air is so dirty, can't drink the tap water because it's so toxic and polluted. Climate change is not part of a conceptual future. It is here. It is now. It is affecting us all, as we continue to witness the proliferation of massive environmental wake-up calls—the loudest we've ever known and experienced—and disproportionately, it's destroying the lives of countless cultures that have perpetuated the *least* amount of ecological damage.

In a growing number of countries, rising sea levels and highly destructive natural disasters are literally killing and uprooting people, devastating life, and obliterating the homes of millions. What once seemed so intangible is now touching the lives of those we know and love in our own backyards—as hurricanes, fires, earthquakes, and floods continue to pick up steam. We have no choice: the time has come to heal, nurture, renew, and inspire real and lasting change for a sustainable and regenerative future for all.

> We have no choice: the time has come to heal, nurture, renew, and inspire real and lasting change for a sustainable and regenerative future for all.

The wonderful thing about the ECOrenaissance is that, in healing our broken world, we only gain, growing exponentially in wisdom, joy, health, and happiness. We find that this movement is not about austerity, deprivation, and sacrifice. It's about love, passion, joy, light, and abundance. It's "yes, and," not "either/or." The idea that this evolution revolution is about depriving yourself comes from the same mind-set that has equated happiness and success with meaningless consumption and waste—at the expense of other human beings and the home we all share. So with equal amounts of urgency and excitement, we actively enter this new chapter of humanity.

Ultimately, individual people will ignite the positive flames of this consciousness renaissance. As isolated individuals we can only do so much, but each of us has the strength and ability to inspire and activate communities, and to harness the power of the collective too. As Margaret Mead so eloquently put it, "Never doubt that a small group of thoughtful, committed citizens can change the world. Indeed, it is the only thing that ever has."[1]

This is the ECOrenaissance—a massive awakening in every corner of the world. We're shaking off the blinders and stepping into the light. We're realizing our true nature, choosing to express rather than repress. We are all powerfully generative, and we crave a world that celebrates authenticity, transparency, creativity, and connectedness.

As we embrace the ECOrenaissance, we're hurtling toward a new normal, where we no longer have to live on the fringes of society to embody a conscious lifestyle. For so many years, things that now have been adopted by the mainstream—eating a plant-based diet, using herbs as medicine, meditating, wearing ECOfashion, and using organic cosmetics—were considered extremely inaccessible and out-there, and most people didn't get the bigger picture of holistic, integrative practice.

When I started my career, I would always say, "I want the norm to be the alternative and the alternative to be the norm." Just two decades later, we're getting there. Change doesn't happen overnight—but sometimes it happens more quickly than you even dream.

> Change doesn't happen overnight—but sometimes it happens more quickly than you even dream.

The train is leaving the station, and it's going only one way. The ECOrenaissance is gaining traction because it's ethical and right in a way that we can feel in our guts—but also because it's exciting and fun. It's about delicious and energizing food; gorgeous fashion and textiles; radiant, lasting beauty; inspiring art; life-changing conversations; and enriched relationships. The more you seek, the more you will find.

I frequently travel for work, and every time I visit a new place I make a point to seek out the local green scene—it's beyond uplifting to see how it's brought to life in different places. And something I have consistently found is that, all over the world, people are speaking a common language. The words may sound different but the message is the same: love, unity, harmony, consciousness, wellness, authenticity, healing, peace. No matter where I am, I feel at home in these communities. There is consistency in this movement all across the world, which constantly excites and motivates me.

Whatever has incited you to take the first step on the ladder of consciousness, take a moment to thank yourself, because the first step is the hardest part. You might not be able to see the top yet, but as you explore each spoke on the wheel of consciousness, embracing the ECOrenaissance community of people who are on the same path to awakening, you climb one step higher, with a greater perspective on what really matters. We are constantly moving forward. In reality, this journey does not end but keeps going as we climb higher and higher, feeling so fulfilled and rewarded every step of the way as we enter a new world and a new normal.

The journey to a sustainable, conscious, thriving, harmonious world begins with individual discoveries. One soul at a time, one day at a time. It starts so small—a whisper of gratitude; a walk in the woods; the pleasure of a local, organic meal with loved ones.

So ignite your light, joining your voice to the ever-growing chorus of movers and shakers who are inspiring beautiful, uplifting change. The time has come to heal, to create, to connect, to inspire. Together we can create a new reality, one that's gorgeous, harmonious, authentic, purpose-driven, and rewarding beyond words. The solutions are clear, and the answers are inside each and every one of us when we really listen. Trust your gut, follow your heart, and live your truth. I invite you to embrace the ECOrenaissance movement and climb the ladder of consciousness with me—I promise, there's a breathtaking view from the top.

If you want to go fast, go alone. If you want to go far, go together.
—AFRICAN PROVERB

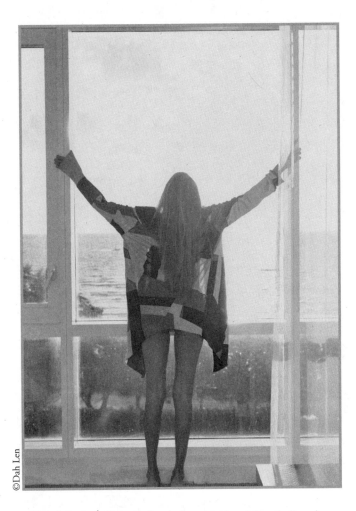

©Dah Len

As I stare blissfully out the window of my 1 Hotel South Beach room in my zero-waste Daniel Silverstein (ZWD) cardigan, I reflect on and embody the deep love and appreciation I feel for the intersection of art, design, nature, and self. This sense of oneness is at the very core of the ECOrenaissance and serves as a reminder to live in the light, where it all begins. Namaste.

Acknowledgments

Having thought of this book concept many years ago, it's been an incredible journey, with every day signifying a rebirth of my true passion and highest self. There are so many people who have helped me make my dreams a reality by contributing their time, wisdom, love, support, and patience.

First and foremost, I'm most grateful to my three greatest sources of light and inspiration: my magnificent daughter Jade Sierra, who is my roommate, best friend, mini-me, and other half of the #greenmore girls. I thank you every day for "getting it." To my extraordinary son Mason Grey, vegan Broadway star in the making, whom I applaud for his humor, tenacity, and for always living his truth; and to my husband, Eric Schnell, twin flame, ECOpreneur partner, and love of my life, with whom I swim in a sea of synchronicity, service, manifestation, and cocreation.

Of course, I owe my very existence to my amazing parents, Jerry and Judy—who taught me the meaning of unconditional love and compassion, and to everyone in my family and extended family—Susan, Rick, Howard, Brenda, my stepchildren Samantha, Ayden, and Colby Schnell, and the Bratmans, Marcovskys, Zaroffs, Fogartys, Davisons, and DiMecos, for celebrating my crazy ideas, supporting my tireless drive, and sharing your love every step of the way. And, of course, I thank my one-of-a-kind uncle, Joe Masteroff, who somehow planted the genetic seed of writing a book. Can't wait to give you a copy.

I can't thank Hazel King enough for showing up in my world at the perfect moment and for assisting me in bringing this book to life. Thanks for keeping me cool and on track when my Sagittarian desire to flow would overtake me. Your raw talent, creative spirit, warm smile, and radiant laughter added so much to the content and positive energy of this book. I am beyond appreciative of Justin Spizman, who has always been there to guide, edit, and support my book process with the utmost integrity, and an unwavering commitment from the very beginning to both me and my vision for this book. I also thank my eco-style sister Sarah Jay for her loving intention, masterful research, and mutual desire to do well by doing good, and both Marlee Book and Danyel Harlem-Siegel for being by my side, ready with beaming vigor, to take on whatever request or challenge is presented.

This book would not be here if it weren't for my visionary Simon & Schuster editor and publisher, Zhena Muzyka of Enliven, who through her own personal path discovered how to heal herself and our global community. A true ECOrenaissance goddess, Zhena believed in me every step of the way and has built an invaluable family of like-minded souls dedicated to the betterment of humanity and the greatest good. And thank you to my wonderful and patient editors, Emily Han and Haley Weaver, and to Judith Curr, founder of Atria, for your unparalleled, game-changing leadership. The publishing world needs more of you.

I also owe huge hugs and gratitude to my über-talented photographer and creative director, Dah Len of *Jack* magazine, for one of my absolute favorite collaborations of all time—at the intersection of Fashion, Art, Soul, and Earth. "FASE" forward, Dah brought to life the most talented and awesome team for my book's photo shoot. The fabulous Danny Santiago brilliantly styled me in clothes from vintage fashion icons to sustainable fashion favorites who graciously shared their eco-chic designs for my shoot, including Stella McCartney, Mara Hoffman, and Daniel Silverstein. Euridice Martin, thank you so much for artfully curating my hair and makeup, even when I was just climbing out of bed at sunrise. Thanks to Kiran Stordalen and Nicole Rechelbacher Thomas of Intelligent Nutrients, Susan Black of EO, Jennifer Rosenberg and Jessica Alba from The Honest Company, and Lauren Singer of The Simply Co, for sharing your incredible products for my shoot, and to masterful jewelry designers Bunny Bedi/Made in Earth and Joanne Stone for loaning your fabulous gemstone and crystal treasures. I'm also extremely grateful to Plant the Future, Simon Dale, Julio Carlos, Sasha Wyroba, Splashlight Studio, Gaby Schuetz, and Alec Diaz for making my South Beach photo shoot so special—our collective efforts demonstrate the magic of cocreation and the convergence of design and nature as a powerful vehicle for positive change.

And an immense thanks to 1 Hotel South Beach—Roxana, Kane, and Raj—for supporting our synergistic vision of a green, chic, and healthy planet. Your stunning eco-resort, and the authentic and symbiotic voice of our mutual connection, served as the most perfect ECOrenaissance home.

To my dear friends and tribe (too many to name), thank you for sharing my journey and for all the love and reinforcement that have fueled my lifework. A special callout to some of my partners and supporters who've been instrumental building blocks along the way, including Joshua Rosenthal, Princess Sarah, Jared Rosen, Anthony Rodale, Dom DeChiara, Fred Neil, Dan and Michelle Jaffe, Scott Greenburg, Romio Shrestha, Walter Robb, John Perkins, Harvey Russack, Pam Rothenberg, Bashar, my teams at Gulliver's, Under the Canopy, MetaWear, BeyondBrands, Good Catch, and Farm to Home, my "THREAD/Driving Fashion Forward" and "AdDRESSing Change" film producing and writing partners Amber Valletta, Amy Johnson, Michelle Vey, Tree Media, and Libby Fearnley, and my Organic Trade Association, Textile Exchange, Fair Trade USA, Cradle to Cradle Innovation Institute, Fashion Revolution, and Aspen Institute Henry Crown Fellowship brothers and sisters.

Thank you to all the "Illuminartists" in and beyond this book who are part of a collective vision to design a positive and prosperous reality for humanity to thrive, and a profound thank-you to my soul family—renowned yogini Surya Little, revolutionary entrepreneur Horst Rechelbacher, and legendary artist Peter Max—who have all played an influential role in my own personal ECOrenaissance.

Life is a blank canvas. Create your own masterpiece. Choose love, light, gratitude, compassion, and consciousness every moment of every day.
—MARCI ZAROFF

Resources

Marci's Food Faves

Alter Eco (www.alterecofoods.com)

Amy's (www.amys.com)

Annie's (www.annies.com)

Califia Farms (www.califiafarms.com)

Clif Bar (www.clifbar.com)

Dean Ornish (www.ornish.com)

Elevation Burger (www.elevationburger.com)

Forks over Knives (www.forksoverknives.com)

Good Catch (www.goodcatchfoods.com)

Good Food Institute (www.gfi.org)

Hilary's Burgers (www.hilaryseatwell.com)

Institute for Integrative Nutrition (www.integrativenutrition.com)

Juice Press (www.juicepress.com)

Just Water (www.justwater.com)

Kevita (www.kevita.com)

Kiss the Ground (www.kisstheground.com)

Liana Werner-Gray/*The Earth Diet* (www.lianawernergray.com)

Living Intentions (www.livingintentions.com)

Living Maxwell (www.livingmaxwell.com)

Mark Hyman (www.drhyman.com)

Miyoko's Kitchen (www.miyokoskitchen.com)

MOM's Organic Market (www.momsorganicmarket.com)

Nature's Path Cereal (www.us.naturespath.com)

Numi Tea (www.numitea.com)

Runa (www.runa.org)

Steaz (www.steaz.com)

Suja Juice (www.sujajuice.com)

Sustainable Food Lab (www.sustainablefoodlab.org)

Thrive Market (www.thrivemarket.com)

Tio Gazpacho (www.tiogazpacho.com)

Whole Foods/365
(www.365bywholefoods.com)

Wicked Healthy
(www.wickedhealthyfood.com)

Marci's Wellness Faves

Chopra Center/Deepak Chopra
(www.deepakchopra.com; www.chopra.com)

Core Power Yoga
(www.corepoweryoga.com)

DailyOM (www.dailyom.com)

Dr. Oz (www.doctoroz.com)

Earthing/grounding (www.earthing.com)

Ecstatic Dance (www.ecstaticdance.org)

Enzymedica (www.enzymedica.com)

Equinox (www.equinox.com)

Exhale (www.exhalespa.com)

Gabrielle Bernstein
(www.gabbybernstein.com)

Gaiam (www.gaiam.com)

Garden of Life (www.gardenoflife.com)

Global Wellness Day
(www.globalwellnessday.org)

Green Spa Network
(www.greenspanetwork.org)

Healthy Child Healthy World/Dr. Harvey
Karp (www.healthychild.org;
www.happiestbaby.com)

Jiyo (www.jiyo.com)

Megafood (www.megafood.com)

Mercola Health Products
(www.mercola.com)

MindBodyGreen
(www.mindbodygreen.com)

New Chapter (www.newchapter.com)

Off the Mat into the World
(www.offthematintotheworld.org)

ORIGIN and *THRIVE* magazines
(www.originmagazine.com;
www.mythrivemag.com)

Pharmaca (www.pharmaca.com)

Soul Cycle (www.soul-cycle.com)

Sustain Condoms
(www.sustainnatural.com)

Tara Stiles/Strala Yoga
(www.tarastiles.com)

Tasha Blank/The Get Down
(www.tashablank.com)

Vitacost (www.vitacost.com)

Well and Good (www.wellandgood.com)

Windmill Health Products
(www.windmillvitamins.com)

XpresSpa (www.xpresspa.com)

Yellow Leaf Hammocks
(www.yellowleafhammocks.com)

Y7 Studio/Hip-Hop Yoga
(www.y7-studio.com)

YogaWorks (www.yogaworks.com)

Marci's Beauty Faves

Acure (www.acureorganics.com)

AVEDA (www.aveda.com)

Bite Lipstick (www.bitebeauty.com)

Credo Beauty (www.credobeauty.com)

Desert Essence (www.desertessence.com)

Dr. Bronner's (www.drbronner.com)

Dr. Hauschka (www.dr.hauschka.com)

EO Products (www.eoproducts.com)

Giovanni (www.giovannicosmetics.com)

Honest Beauty/Jessica Alba
(www.honestbeauty.com)

Hynt Beauty (www.hyntbeauty.com)

I AM fragrance (www.iamfragrance.com)

Indie Beauty Expo
(www.indiebeautyexpo.com)

Intelligent Nutrients
(www.intelligentnutrients.com)

Josie Maran
(www.josiemarancosmetics.com)

Kristen Arnett Makeup Artist
(www.kristenarnett.com)

Lotus Wei (www.lotuswei.com)

Not Just a Pretty Face
(www.notjustaprettyface.org)

RMS (www.rmsbeauty.com)

Skin Deep/EWG (www.EWG.org/skindeep)

Tarte Cosmetics (www.tartecosmetics.com)

Tata Harper (www.tataharper.com)

Marci's Fashion Faves

Able Made (www.ablemadeshop.com)

About Organic Cotton
(www.aboutorganiccotton.org)

AWEAR World/Kestrel Jenkins
(www.awearworld.com)

Bead & Reel (www.beadandreel.com)

BFDA (www.bkaccelerator.com)

C&A Foundation
(www.candafoundation.org)

Canopy Planet (www.canopyplanet.org)

Common Objective
(www.commonobjective.co)

Copenhagen Fashion Summit
(www.copenhagenfashionsummit.com)

Coyuchi (www.coyuchi.com)

Daniel Silverstein
(www.zerowastedaniel.com)

ECOcult/Alden Wicker (www.ecocult.com)

ECOfashion Talk/Sass Brown
(www.ecofashiontalk.com)

EcoSalon (www.ecosalon.com)

Eco Warrior Princess
(www.ecowarriorprincess.net)

Eileen Fisher (www.eileenfisher.com)

Emma Watson (www.emma-watson.net)

Etsy (www.etsy.com)

Fair Fashion Center at Glasgow Caledonian
University (www.gcufairfashioncenter.org)

Farm to Home (www.farmtohomeorganic
.com)

Fashion Heroes (www.fashionheroes.eco)

Fashion Me Green/Greta Eagan
(www.fashionmegreen.com)

Fashion Positive (www.fashionpositive.org)

Fashion Revolution Day
(www.fashionrevolution.org)

Fashion Takes Action
(www.fashiontakesaction.org)

FEED Projects (www.feedprojects.com)

Fibershed (www.fibershed.com)

Green Carpet Challenge
(www.eco-age.com/green-carpet-challenge)

Green Shows (www.thegreenshows.com)

Grund America (www.grundamerica.com)

H&M (www.hm.com)

Helpsy (www.shophelpsy.com)

I-CO (www.ico-spirit.com)

Indigenous (www.indigenous.com)

Inhabitat (formerly Ecouterre)
(www.inhabitat.com)

Joanne Stone Jewelry
(www.joannestonedesign.com)

Kaight (www.kaightshop.com)

Kering (www.kering.com)

Lenzing Fibers (www.lenzing.com)

Live the Process (www.livetheprocess.com)

Livia Firth/Eco Age (www.eco-age.com)

Lux & Eco (www.luxandeco.com)

Made in Earth Jewelry
(www.madeinearthus.com)

Magnifeco/Kate Black
(www.magnifeco.com)

Maiyet (www.maiyet.com)

Maker's Row (www.makersrow.com)

Mara Hoffman (www.marahoffman.com)

MetaWear (www.metawearorganic.com)

Modavanti (www.modavanti.com)

MUD Jeans (www.mudjeans.eu)

Naturepedic Mattresses
(www.naturepedic.com)

Nau (www.nau.com)

Nineteenth Amendment
(www.nineteenthamendment.com)

Outerknown (www.outerknown.com)

PACT (www.wearpact.com)

Parley for the Oceans
(www.parleyfortheoceans.com)

Patagonia (www.patagonia.com)

People Tree (www.peopletree.co.uk)

Prana (www.prana.com)

Recover (www.recovertex.com)

Red Carpet Green Dress
(www.redcarpetgreendress.com)

Redress/Christina Dean
(www.redress.com.hk)

Reformation (www.thereformation.com)

Renewal Workshop
(www.renewalworkshop.com)

Rent the Runway
(www.renttherunway.com)

Reve en Vert (www.reve-en-vert.com)

Satya Jewelry (www.satyajewelry.com)

Shop Ethica (www.shopethica.com)

SITO (www.mercola.com)

Soko Jewelry (www.shopsoko.com)

Stella McCartney
(www.stellamccartney.com)

Studio 189/Rosario Dawson
(www.studiooneeightynine.com)

Sustainable Apparel Coalition
(www.apparelcoalition.org)

Sustainably Chic
(www.sustainably-chic.com)

Textile Exchange (www.textileexchange.org)

Thread: A Documentary (www
.threaddocumentary.com)

TOMS Shoes (www.toms.com)

The True Cost (www.truecostmovie.com)

Under the Canopy
(www.underthecanopy.com)

Vandana Shiva (www.vandanashiva.com)

Warby Parker (www.warbyparker.com)

Zady (www.zady.com)

Marci's Conscious Business Faves

ABC Home/Paulette Cole
(www.abchome.com)

Airbnb (www.airbnb.com)

American Sustainable Business Council
(www.asbcouncil.org)

Apple (www.apple.com)

B Corp (www.bcorporation.net)

BeyondBrands (www.beyondbrands.org)

Conscious Commerce
(www.consciousco.co)

ECOS (www.ecos.com)

FounderMade (www.foundermade.com)

GreenBiz (www.greenbiz.com)

Lexus/Toyota (www.lexus.com/hybrid)

LinkedIn for Good
(www.linkedinforgood.linkedin.com)

Method (www.methodhome.com)

Near Future Summit
(www.nearfuturesummit.com)

1 Hotels (www.1hotels.com)

Seventh Generation
(www.seventhgeneration.com)

Starbucks (www.starbucks.com)

Summit Series (www.summit.co)

Sustainable Brands International
(www.sustainablebrands.com)

Target (www.corporate.target.com)

Tesla/Elon Musk (www.tesla.com)

Unilever (Sustainable Living Platform)
(www.unilever.com)

Virgin Group/Richard Branson
(www.virgin.com)

More of Marci's Faves: VIPs/Causes/Media/Thought Leaders/Events

Abraham Hicks (www.abraham-hicks.com)

Adrian Grenier (www.adriangrenier.com)

Alan Watts (www.alanwatts.org)

Amazon Watch (www.amazonwatch.org)

Aspen Institute (www.aspeninstitute.org)

Bashar (www.bashar.org)

Biomimicry/Janine Benyus
(www.biomimicry.org)

Burning Man (www.burningman.org)

BuzzFeed (www.buzzfeed.com)

Captain Planet Foundation
(www.captainplanetfoundation.org)

Center for Food Safety
(www.centerforfoodsafety.org)

Climate Reality Project
(www.climaterealityproject.org)

Cradle to Cradle (www.c2ccertified.org)

Debbie Ford (www.debbieford.com)

Do Something (www.dosomething.org)

Dr. Gabrielle Francis
(www.theherbanalchemist.com)

Elephant Journal
(www.elephantjournal.com)

Entertainment for Change
(www.entertainmentforchange.com)

Environmental Working Group
(www.ewg.org)

Envision Festival
(www.envisionfestival.com)

Every Mother Counts/Christy Turlington (www.everymothercounts.org)

Evolver Network (www.evolver.net)

Fair Labor Association (www.fairlabor.org)

Fair Trade USA (www.fairtradeusa.org)

5 Gyres Institute (www.5gyres.org)

Global Green USA (www.globalgreen.org)

GOOP/Gwyneth Paltrow (www.goop.com)

Graham Hancock (www.grahamhancock.com)

Gregg Braden (www.greggbraden.com)

Huffington Post (www.huffingtonpost.com)

Humane Society (www.humanesociety.org)

Jack Johnson (www.jackjohnsonmusic.com)

Jason Mraz (www.jasonmraz.com)

Jason Silva (www.thisisjasonsilva.com)

Joe Rogan (www.joerogan.net)

John Hardy/*Green by John* blog (www.GreenbyJohn.com)

John Perkins/Dream Change (www.johnperkins.org; www.dreamchange.org)

Kahlil Gibran (www.gibrankhalilgibran.org)

Leonardo DiCaprio (www.leonardodicaprio.com; www.beforetheflood.com)

Marianne Williamson (www.marianne.com)

Mark Ruffalo (markruffalo.tumblr.com)

Mercy for Animals (www.mercyforanimals.org)

Moby (www.moby.com)

Ms. Foundation (www.forwomen.org)

Natural Resources Defense Council (www.NRDC.org)

Nature Conservancy (www.nature.org)

Neil DeGrasse Tyson (www.haydenplanetarium.org/tyson)

NowThis (www.nowthisnews.com)

Oceana (www.oceana.org)

1 Billion Rising (www.onebillionrising.org)

Operation Warm (www.operationwarm.org)

Oprah Winfrey (www.oprah.com)

Organic Authority (www.organicauthority.com)

Organic Center for Research & Promotion (www.organic-center.org)

Organic Consumers Association (www.organicconsumers.org)

Organic Trade Association (www.ota.com)

PETA (People for the Ethical Treatment of Animals) (www.peta.org)

Peter Max (www.petermax.com)

Rainforest Alliance (www.rainforest-alliance.org)

Rainforest Foundation/Sting/Trudie (www.rainforestfoundation.org)

Refinery 29 (www.refinery29.com)

Renaissance Human
(www.renaissancehuman.co)

Resonance Project/Nassim Haramein
(www.theconnecteduniversefilm.com;
www.resonance.is)

Rodale Institute/Maria Rodale
(www.rodale.com; www.rodaleinstitute.org)

Russell Brand (www.russellbrand.com)

SEED Food & Wine Week
(www.seedfoodandwine.com)

Senator Cory Booker
(www.corybooker.com)

Shailene Woodley
(www.twitter.com/shailenewoodley)

ShiftCon (www.shiftconmedia.com)

South by Southwest (www.sxsw.com)

Spirit Science (www.thespiritscience.net)

Susan Rockefeller
(www.protectwhatisprecious.com)

TED Talks/TEDx (www.ted.com/talks)

Textile Exchange (www.textileexchange.org)

The Assemblage (www.theassemblage.com)

The Solutions Project
(www.thesolutionsproject.org)

Thrive Movement/Foster Gamble
(www.thrivemovement.com)

Turning Green (www.turninggreen.org)

UC Berkeley Haas Business School
(www.haas.berkeley.edu)

Upworthy (www.upworthy.com)

Van Jones (www.vanjones.net)

Vice Media (www.vice.com)

Wanderlust (www.wanderlust.com)

Women's Business Enterprise
(www.wbenc.org)

Women's Prison Association
(www.wpaonline.org)

Notes

Introduction

1 Shakti Gawain, *Living in the Light: Follow Your Inner Guidance to Create a New Life and a New World* (Novato, CA: New World Library, 1986).

About the Book

1 Hendrick Willem van Loon, *The Story of Mankind* (New York: Liveright/W. W. Norton, updated edition 2013).

1: The Five Cs of the ECOrenaissance Movement

1 HeartMath Institute, "Science of the Heart," https://www.heartmath.org/research/science-of-the -heart/.
2 Rollin McCraty, PhD; Annette Deyhle, PhD; and Doc Childre, "The Global Coherence Initiative: Creating a Coherent Planetary Standing Wave," *Global Advances in Health and Medicine* 1, no. 1 (2012): 64–77, https://www.ncbi.nlm.nih.gov/pmc/articles/PMC3833489/.

2: Life Is Art

1 Ross Andersen, "A Timothy Leary for the Viral Video Age," *Atlantic*, April 12, 2012, https://www .theatlantic.com/technology/archive/2012/04/a-timothy-leary-for-the-viral-video-age/255691/.
2 Susan Daugherty, "DJ Spooky: Multimedia Mixes to Save the Planet," *National Geographic*, October 30, 2014, https://news.nationalgeographic.com/news/2014/10/141030-emerging-explorer-miller -spooky-art-antarctica-climate-change-music/.
3 Burning Man, "The 10 Principles of Burning Man," https://burningman.org/culture/philosophical -center/10-principles/.
4 Creative Bloq, "10 Digital Artists You Need to Know About," http://www.creativebloq.com/digital-art /10-digital-artists-you-need-know-11618947.
5 Beyoncé, "Beygood to Mother Earth," https://www.beyonce.com/free-ways-to-be-green-earth-day -beyonce/.

6 Kathy Freston, "The Breathtaking Effects of Cutting Back on Meat," *Huffington Post*, May 2, 2009 (updated November 17, 2011), https://www.huffingtonpost.com/kathy-freston/the-breathtaking -effects_b_181716.html.

7 Ibid.

3: Evolved Epicure

1 OEHHA, "Glyphosate Listed Effective July 7, 2017, as Known to the State of California to Cause Cancer," https://oehha.ca.gov/proposition-65/crnr/glyphosate-listed-effective-july-7-2017-known -state-california-cause-cancer.

2 Marla Cone, "New Study: Autism Linked to Environment," *Scientific American*, January 9, 2009, https://www.scientificamerican.com/article/autism-rise-driven-by-environment/.

3 GMO FAQ, "Where Are GMOs Grown and Banned?" https://gmo.geneticliteracyproject.org/FAQ /where-are-gmos-grown-and-banned/.

4 Larry Kopald, presentation, Regeneration International Conference, San Miguel de Allende, Mexico, October 2017.

5 Organic Trade Association, "Millennials and Organic: A Winning Combination," https://www.ota .com/news/press-releases/19256.

6 Nielsen, "Organic Products Are Showing Up in More Places—and for Less Money," http://www .nielsen.com/us/en/insights/news/2017/organic-products-are-showing-up-in-more-places-and-for-less -money.html.

7 The Carbon Underground and Regenerative Agriculture Initiative, "What Is Regenerative Agriculture?" February 24, 2017, http://regenerationinternational.org/2017/02/24/what-is-regenerative-agriculture/.

8 Kiss the Ground, https://kisstheground.com/.

9 One Green Planet, "Facts on Animal Farming and the Environment," http://www.onegreenplanet.org /animalsandnature/facts-on-animal-farming-and-the-environment/.

10 Jordyn Cormier, "Which Is Worse for the Planet: Beef or Cars?" *EcoWatch*, July 13, 2016, https://www .ecowatch.com/which-is-worse-for-the-planet-beef-or-cars-1919932136.html.

11 One Green Planet, "Milk Life? How About Milk Destruction: The Shocking Truth About the Dairy Industry and the Environment," http://www.onegreenplanet.org/animalsandnature/the-dairy-industry -and-the-environment/.

12 World Wildlife Fund, https://www.worldwildlife.org/industries/dairy/.

13 David Biello, "Overfishing Could Take Seafood off the Menu by 2048," *Scientific American*, November 2, 2006, https://www.scientificamerican.com/article/overfishing-could-take-se/.

14 WWF, "Farmed Seafood: Overview," https://www.worldwildlife.org/industries/farmed-seafood.

15 Ibid.

16 Wicked Healthy Food, https://www.wickedhealthyfood.com/about/.

17 Virginia I. Lohr, "What Are the Benefits of Plants Indoors and Why Do We Respond Positively to Them?" Department of Horticulture and Landscape Architecture, 1996, https://public.wsu.edu/~lohr /pub/2010LohrBenefitsPltsIndoors.pdf.

18 Brian Fung, "How 40% of Our Food Goes to Waste," *Atlantic*, August 23, 2012, https://www .theatlantic.com/health/archive/2012/08/how-40-of-our-food-goes-to-waste/261498/.

19 CNN, "40% of U.S. Food Wasted, Report Says," CNN blog, August 22, 2012, http://news.blogs.cnn
.com/2012/08/22/40-of-u-s-food-wasted-report-says/.

20 Maura Judkis, "The Simple Labeling Update That Could Prevent Millions of Tons of Food from
Going in the Trash," *Washington Post*, May 19, 2016, https://www.washingtonpost.com/news/food/wp
/2016/05/19/the-simple-labeling-update-that-could-prevent-millions-of-tons-of-food-from-going-in
-the-trash/?utm_term=.957a28063e56.

4: It's All Well and Good

1 *Science Daily*, "Top Water Saving Tips for American Households," https://www.sciencedaily.com
/releases/2014/07/140729101130.htm.

2 Sue Thomas, "Gazing at Virtual Nature Is Good for Your Psychological Well-being," *Slate*, December
17, 2013, http://www.slate.com/blogs/future_tense/2013/12/17/nearby_nature_effect_biophilic
_design_looking_at_virtual_trees_is_good_for.html.

3 Danielle Posa, *Wellbeing Hacker*, https://www.wellbeinghacker.com.

4 Sustainable Furnishings Council, https://sustainablefurnishings.org/.

5 Dan Buettner, *The Blue Zones: Lessons for Living Longer from the People Who've Lived the Longest*
(Washington, DC: National Geographic, 2008).

6 Harvard Health Publishing, "Drugs in the Water," https://www.health.harvard.edu/newsletter_article
/drugs-in-the-water.

7 The Earthing Institute, "What Is Earthing?" http://www.earthinginstitute.net/what-is-earthing/.

8 Armin Rosen, "The Science Behind Mindfulness and Meditation," *Huffington Post*, July 14,
2017, http://www.huffingtonpost.com/entry/the-science-behind-mindfulness-and-meditation_us
_59677a0de4b07b5e1d96eda1.

9 Deborah Bloom, "Instead of Detention, These Students Get Meditation," CNN, November 8, 2016,
http://www.cnn.com/2016/11/04/health/meditation-in-schools-baltimore/index.html.

5: Beauty Inside and Out

1 Environmental Defence, "Report: Pre-Polluted," http://environmentaldefence.ca/report/report-pre
-polluted-a-report-on-toxic-substances-in-the-umbilical-cord-blood-of-canadian-newborns/.

2 Adria Vasil, *Ecoholic Body: Your Ultimate Earth-Friendly Guide to Living Healthy and Looking Good*
(Montreal: Vintage, 2012).

3 State of California Environmental Protection Agency, Office of Environmental Health Hazard
Assessment, "Chemicals Known to the State to Cause Cancer or Reproductive Toxicity," December 29,
2017, https://oehha.ca.gov/media/downloads/proposition-65//p65122917.pdf.

4 Lenny Letter, "Alicia Keys: Time to Uncover," accessed October 29, 2017, http://www.lennyletter.com
/style/a410/alicia-keys-time-to-uncover/.

5 Laura Capon, "Alicia Keys Has Stopped Wearing Makeup and Is Killing It," *Cosmopolitan*, November
21, 2016.

6 Naomi Wolf, *The Beauty Myth: How Images of Beauty Are Used Against Women* (New York:
HarperCollins, 2002).

6: Styling Change

1 Heidy Rehman, "Shocking Environmental Implications of Fashion," *Huffington Post*, August 19, 2016, http://www.huffingtonpost.co.uk/heidy-rehman/shocking-environmental-fast-fashion_b_8009850 .html.

2 Organic Consumer Association, "Care What You Wear: Facts on Cotton & Clothing Production," https://www.organicconsumers.org/news/care-what-you-wear-facts-cotton-clothing-production.

3 Ibid.

4 Claire Meeghan, "Pesticide Poisoning: Confronting the Hidden Menace," *Guardian*, August 2, 2013, https://www.theguardian.com/global-development/poverty-matters/2013/aug/02/pesticide-poisoning -hidden-menace-ghana.

5 Rodale Institute, "About Us: The History of Rodale Institute," https://rodaleinstitute.org/about-us /mission-and-history/.

6 GOOP, "A Q&A with Marci Zaroff," http://goop.com/wellness/food-planet/is-your-clothing-toxic/.

7 http://www.greenpeace.org/international/en/campaigns/detox/.

8 https://echa.europa.eu/.

9 https://www.chemicalsafetyfacts.org/.

10 Textile Exchange, presentation, Textile Exchange Annual Conference and Reports, Potomac, MD, October 2017.

11 Sarah Maisey, "Style Meets Sustainability at the Green Carpet Fashion Awards in Milan," *National*, October 1, 2017, https://www.thenational.ae/lifestyle/fashion/style-meets-sustainability-at-the-green -carpet-fashion-awards-in-milan-1.663072.

12 United Nations, "Transforming Our World: the 2030 Agenda for Sustainable Development," https:// sustainabledevelopment.un.org/post2015/transformingourworld.

13 Andrew Brown and Jane Hutchison, eds., *Organising Labour in Globalising Asia* (London: Routledge, 2001); John Hilary, *The Poverty of Capitalism: Economic Meltdown and the Struggle for What Comes Next* (London: Pluto Press, 2013).

14 Safia Minney, keynote address, World Ethical Apparel Roundtable (WEAR) 2016, hosted by Fashion Takes Action, Toronto.

15 Tansy Hoskins, "Reliving the Rana Plaza Factory Collapse: A History of Cities in 50 Buildings, Day 22," *Guardian*, April 23, 2015, https://www.theguardian.com/cities/2015/apr/23/rana-plaza-factory -collapse-history-cities-50-buildings.

16 A Bull's-eye View, "Sustainability," https://corporate.target.com/corporate-responsibility /sustainability.

17 Teslin Doud, speech, Copenhagen Fashion Summit, Copenhagen, May 2017.

7: Conscious Business and Consumerism

1 Andrew Winston, *The Big Pivot: Radically Practical Strategies for a Hotter, Scarcer, and More Open World* (Boston: Harvard Business Review Press, 2014).

2 Author email interview with Andrew Winston, October 17, 2017.

3 Dream Change, "Why the Love Summit?" https://www.dreamchange.org/the-love-summit/.
4 Ibid.
5 Howard Thurman Center for Common Ground, "History," https://www.bu.edu/thurman/about/history/.

Conclusion

1 Nancy C. Lutkehaus, *Margaret Mead: The Making of an American Icon* (Princeton, NJ: Princeton University Press, 2008).